Life on a Knife's Edge

Life on a Knife's Edge

A Brain Surgeon's Reflections on Life, Loss and Survival

RAHUL JANDIAL

PENGUIN LIFE

AN IMPRINT OF

PENGUIN BOOKS

PENGUIN LIFE

UK | USA | Canada | Ireland | Australia
India | New Zealand | South Africa

Penguin Life is part of the Penguin Random House group of companies
whose addresses can be found at global.penguinrandomhouse.com.

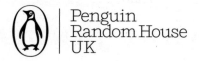

First published 2021
001

Copyright © Rahul Jandial, 2021

The moral right of the author has been asserted

Set in 13.5/16pt Dante MT Std
Typeset by Jouve (UK), Milton Keynes
Printed and bound in Great Britain by Clays Ltd, Elcograf S.p.A.

The authorized representative in the EEA is Penguin Random House Ireland,
Morrison Chambers, 32 Nassau Street, Dublin D02 YH68

A CIP catalogue record for this book is available from the British Library

HARDBACK ISBN: 978–0–241–46182–2
TRADE PAPERBACK ISBN: 978–0–241–46183–9

www.greenpenguin.co.uk

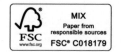

For my sons
Zain, Kai, Ronak

Contents

Preface

When I began writing this book, my goal was to pull back the blue surgical drapes and give an insider's view of brain surgery. My intention was to reveal what really happens after the patients are lying on the table in the operating theatre, their brains exposed and glistening. And what happens when they wake up and come to terms with their altered lives.

The resulting book is something quite different. I realized I could not write honestly about my experiences in surgery without pulling back the curtain on myself, to expose myself in the same level of detail and depth as my patients.

I am a brain cancer surgeon. I'm also a neurobiologist leading research that will, I hope, one day make my operating skills unnecessary through advancements in science. But, for now, I remove cancer from people. A lot. I'm good at what I do, but the very nature of my work means I often fail.

I have extended thousands of lives. I have outflanked death on the operating table many times. I have given people those extra months of life so they can see their children graduate. I have also inflicted terrible pain that could have been avoided. I have made mistakes that have haunted me for years. I have made decisions that have saved lives. I've made others I'm proud of that pushed the boundaries of professional ethics and could have ended my career.

I have never seen myself as above the law, but when I was taking care of patients with severe brain injuries I was often placed in impossible scenarios that very few could ever imagine. There are compromises that have to be made, awful, unavoidable choices that surgeons and patients sometimes have to face.

Surgeons have the reputation of being more interested in the procedure than the person. I never saw it that way. For me, surgery was never about human anatomy but about human nature. I am indebted to the craft of surgery, a practice that lays bare both my patient and me, placing us both on a knife's edge. It can be a lonely place and there are rarely any easy answers.

The questions that we face in surgery are the biggest ones conceivable, reaching deep into the heart of what it is to be sentient, aware – an attempt to investigate the wonder of the human mind. And what deeper connection can there be between two humans than one permitting the other to cut them open and work inside them? And in my particular specialty, the patient may even be conscious while I perform the brain surgery. One mind inside another.

The journeys I have been on with my patients have been a masterclass in the fragility, courage and beauty of humanity. And to care for the suffering, I have had to bring my own suffering to the fore. What I share in the following pages is my personal foray into the ethics and struggles that my patients and I have experienced.

In this book I share the lessons and insights from the trenches of my life and my work, everything my patients have taught me about our remarkable brains and the precious life we have. I am forever indebted to them. My patients have taught me grace, courage and true wisdom out of their most trying circumstances, and have made me think differently about life, loss and survival. In the pages that follow, I share what I have learned.

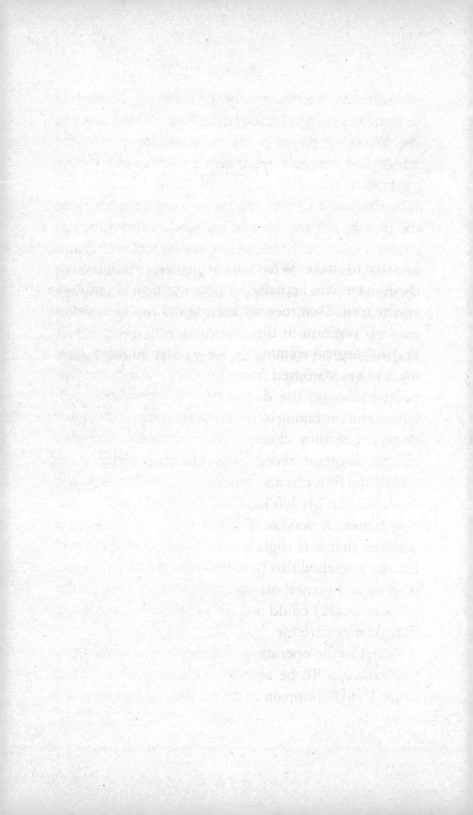

Trauma

I started to shake. What felt like an early inkling of an earthquake was actually a helicopter touching down on the roof. That meant I had about sixty seconds to get into position in the trauma bay. It was my first year in surgical training. A woman hit by stray gunfire had been airlifted from 'the field'. When she was rushed through the doors, her blood pressure collapsed and the falling numbers pulsing on the monitor showed just how close to death she was. The lead trauma surgeon sliced between the woman's left fourth and fifth ribs and told me to literally pump her heart for her. My left hand barely fitted between the two bones; it was as if I was reaching through a window that was slightly ajar. I was wrist deep and felt the stretched ribs bow back snugly on my wrist. And when I turned my hand to grab the base of the slippery heart I could feel her ribs splinter and crack to accommodate me.

To get to the operating theatre, we had to navigate the hallways. To be able to continue clenching her heart, I had to jump on to the gurney. We were rushed so hard through the sharp turns that sometimes I was not only squeezing her heart, I had to hold on to it to keep from losing my grip. I could feel her warm blood on my forearm. The muscles in my hand cramped as I held her heart in my palm. Squeezing. Then releasing. An open cardiac massage was a rare surgical manoeuvre, performed when a patient has lost more than half their blood and the heart fails to pump; there is too little to fill it, so it merely flutters.

When we reached the operating room, two surgeons were waiting. Without a word, the surgeon pushed me away from the patient with his elbow. I stumbled backwards and my hand slid out of her, releasing her heart. That was his intention. Then he and the other surgeon took over. They incised, dissected and found the sheared arteries in her chest and abdomen while two anaesthesiologists plunged blood and medicines into her veins.

In four hours of orchestrated chaos, they worked frenetically but in unison, and the patient lived. It was the most powerful thing I had ever witnessed, a scene that is unimaginable to the uninitiated. What made it even more incredible was how unlikely it was I was there in the first place. Six years earlier, I'd been a college dropout. At that moment I felt deeply proud of the craft I had entered, and the word 'surgery' took on new depth. I had seen surgeons perform together, and at the highest level.

I wanted more.

Today, I'm a brain surgeon specializing in removing cancer from people's bodies. Now in my forties, I've met more than fifteen thousand patients and operated on more than four thousand. Surgery can inflict damage on the most human aspects of ourselves but also reveal our deepest humanity.

As a surgeon in training, I experienced something else entirely. Work on the general trauma service goes down at a different pace. If your body is shattered by a gunshot, a car accident or some other catastrophe, you don't wait in line to be seen. You are sent directly to a trauma bay. With your clothes on, it's hard to tell how torn you are. We don't gently slip off your trousers. A trauma shear is run up each leg until it cuts through the waistline. Your shirt is also split in two. Minimal movement for the broken body lying there. Nudity is not a concern. Get to the access points. Look for any open fractures. Get to the ribs. Be ready to make holes to let trapped air out. All of this to stop you, the patient, from hitting the ground if you're spiralling downwards. You are hurtling towards a hard and cold earth, and this is the last point the parachute can be activated. Surgeons are your last hope to pull you out of this nosedive.

A few days after I held that woman's heart in my hand, I was back in the trauma bay, helping to handle a deluge of patients. I stood looking at the scene in front of me and remembered something I'd locked away from my past. The clothes of several patients which I had sheared off and had not yet been swept away looked like leaves raked into a pile, a mass of shapes, hues and textures. Their shoes had been discarded at the site of the motorway pile-up, giving an air of incompleteness to the shredded wardrobe of garments.

The remnants of their clothing triggered something in my peripheral vision. It seems that's how I notice things. We don't have a blind spot in our peripheral vision. There, I saw a bizarre kaleidoscopic Rorschach blot. At that moment, something came to mind; something I had seen over the skies of Los Angeles when I was thirteen years old but had tucked away.

The Los Angeles basin encompasses 13 million people and more than 4,500 square miles, stretching out in every direction and limited only by the Pacific Ocean. Inside the metropolis is a completely forgettable city called Cerritos. One Sunday in August 1986 I was out riding my bike. It was then that I heard the sound. It was subtle at first, but unforgettable, because it had an unfamiliar amplitude and frequency. Clearly metallic and explosive, but quite distant. I looked left and right to see where it was coming from. Nothing. Then I looked up. The sound had escalated into a weird screeching, a million fingernails scratching a chalkboard.

As I rode closer, I remember vividly that there were no shadows, no ghost bicycle with spinning wheels that usually accompanied me on one side or the other. The sun was directly above me. Noon. The sight of a passenger jet careening in the air, dangling from its tail like a Christmas ornament, left no doubt what was happening and what was about to happen.

The soul-shaking thud was actually a relief after the sound of the screaming jet engines. The pieces rained on Carmenita Road in Cerritos, the main road that led to my home, my school and the overpass that was my vantage point. I saw torn pieces of clothes, like falling autumn leaves. The clothes on the trauma bay floor had unlocked this memory: witnessing the aftermath of a single-engine plane colliding with an Aeroméxico flight on approach to Los Angeles International Airport over Cerritos.

Back then, an aeroplane crash didn't carry the immediate assumptions and triggers it does now, after 9/11. Back then, also, the little city didn't have the understanding and foresight to block off the wreckage, as municipalities do now. I got disconcertingly close. The smell of fuel was brand new. Not like the smell of burning I was used to but a unique blend of molten plastic and metal. And then, beneath the fuel, something I would smell again many years later. Burning flesh. My brain didn't know where to place it. A first exposure. Later, when I became a surgeon, the smell would become familiar to me.

The memory floated up to the front of my brain, the place where cognition and emotion mix, unexpected and unbidden. The human brain is like a dense forest canopy, with conscious thought – the cognitive brain – in the treetops and the emotion of the visceral brain in the branches all converging down towards the trunk – the reptilian brainstem. The memory had risen up from the interacting elements of this concealed space.

We are the sum of our memories. They shape our understanding of the world, connecting us to our past and the people closest to us. Memories can also be our undoing. Most traumatic memories fade, their sharp edges dulled by time. When they remain undiminished, however, they can haunt us. They can disrupt our daily lives, making us unable to focus or function. These intrusive memories germinate after trauma, sprouting and growing pernicious roots. Like some unwanted and malevolent visitor from the past, they arrive uninvited and do not let us forget. The way we deal with these traumatic memories is vital, because we're unlikely to make it through life without avoiding trauma entirely.

Experiencing trauma is a by-product of the human condition. Most of us have had or will have a traumatic event in our lives. For many of us, it will be multiple traumas. The best estimates suggest that roughly three quarters of people worldwide have experienced at least one traumatic event. We've witnessed a death or a grave injury, been assaulted, suffered a life-threatening illness or experienced the unexpected death of a loved one.

I've seen the body hurt in every unimaginable way. Trauma leaves its survivors permanently altered. They are physically altered, of course, forced to move forward with new, damaged bodies. But they are also psychologically altered, and recovering from the emotional scar of a traumatic event is often harder than physical rehabilitation.

After severe trauma, patients are usually unconscious when they are brought into hospital. They come without identification, and their family members are still unaware of what's taken place. For these patients in the US, we have the right as surgeons to invoke a process we call 'double doc' – one doctor makes the plan; a second doctor consents – which means we don't need your consent to save your life. We rescue you in ways you may have found objectionable had you been conscious.

When a trauma victim wakes up, it's already happened: ribs sliced, bowels rerouted, brain lobes removed, limbs amputated. At first, they are often groggy and not fully aware. The mix of narcotics and the realization that they have survived is almost always met with relief, even by some who attempted suicide. They don't have the foresight to know the long journey ahead to becoming physically independent and free from the aftershocks of what they've been through.

Once they are out of the intensive care unit (ICU) or on lower doses of drugs, I begin to see differences in people. And it's not just about whether they have social support systems or resources. It's about whether a poisonous emotion takes hold – guilt. If what happened was out of their control, the patients are thankful to be alive and direct their emotions and their grief outwards, to fate, to someone or something else, but rarely inwards, at themselves. However, if it was an error in their judgement that led to the trauma – for example, they hadn't been wearing a seat belt – patients struggle with inwardly directed guilt and shame, a sense that 'I did this to myself.'

These days patients set an appointment to see me in clinic, and surgery is mostly scheduled. Most of my patients have not survived a trauma but are in the middle of one. Being told they have cancer is a trauma in itself. Some hear the diagnosis in a hospital bed. They aren't in the professional clothes they don for a clinic visit, but stripped down, essential, in just a thin hospital gown. No clothes, rings, watch. My patients have malignant brain and spinal tumours that invariably grow back. Often, the surgery provides the diagnosis.

When preparing to tell the patient what I've found, I usually go to the side of the bed that forces them to look away from the door and towards me. Looking at the door is a classic dodge for patients who wish to avoid what they are about to hear. They become distracted, no doubt imagining escape from the bed, the hospital, the news coming their way. Perhaps strangely, I found that trauma in my own life had primed me to be able to help patients under existential threat from a brain tumour or other life-threatening conditions.

I give patients the news with an expression I hope conveys both that I'm sure what I'm saying is true and that it hurts me to have to say it: 'It is – cancer.' And then I'm quiet. One or two minutes of silence usually follow; the patient needs this time to register the collapse in their world, and to pilot their thoughts and emotions, layered and coloured by who they are, about what they have been through, what they may have thought about a cancer diagnosis, and who they are responsible for. That 'life flashing before your eyes' thing doesn't happen in your last seconds while you drift towards the proverbial white light. It happens when you hear the word 'cancer'. I can see the patient's breathing change, the lines of their face shift; most react with pain and tears.

When I see they are braced, I start pulling them out of their free fall. I tell them the months ahead are theirs, but not the decades. No cure exists. I tell them we can work to get years. Pain-free years. Precious years. I promise to take them through as much of it as they want me to. Unlike with a car crash or a heart attack, the emotional pain of a cancer diagnosis doesn't relent, it evolves.

With treatment comes another form of trauma. Surgery, chemotherapy and radiation therapy can bring pain, discomfort and bodily changes. As hard as that is, however, the emotional pain of cancer may be worse. Women with a type of localized breast cancer that gave them a better than 90 per cent survival rate found the most stressful experiences had nothing to do with their treatment. They were, in descending order: having a physician inform you of a cancer diagnosis; waiting for the results of the surgery to see if the cancer has spread; and the waiting period prior to the cancer surgery.

For some brain cancer patients, there is no escaping their destiny. They have to quickly adjust to seeing their mortality in sharp focus. The finish line of their lives is suddenly thrust into view. Immediately, they want to push it back. Do whatever they need to do to have a chance at more months, more years. The patient barely has time to recover from one treatment before bracing themselves for the next test results and the treatments they may bring. To me, that's heroism: getting up in the morning and going to the cancer centre against the odds, and in spite of them.

My trauma patients get caught up in a storm, while my cancer patients ask to be taken into the storm. It's a completely different experience. Later, as the cancer treatments take their toll and only palliative options remain, the patient suffers a different trauma. Dying. Not death. They worry their dying will not be dignified.

How we digest trauma over time can make all the

difference. It is possible for most of us to endure life's physical and emotional traumas without developing crippling symptoms. The risk of a traumatic event causing a severe and long-lasting reaction is increased by how close we are to the trauma physically and emotionally, and how we choose to respond to it.

Coping strategies that work in the short run can become toxic. Walling off the trauma in our minds in the immediate aftermath keeps it from overwhelming us, but the injury can come back in unexpected and harmful ways. This mimics what happens in the brain when the skull is violated by a blow. If you're struck by a hammer or fall on your head, the flesh of your brain reacts immediately at a cellular level. Neurons are surrounded by allies called glia, which protect them so the injury doesn't spread to neighbouring healthy neurons, like falling dominoes. Like the neurons themselves, these glia are precious. Their response to an injury, the way they surround and protect the neurons, is called gliosis. It looks like a scar, visible to the naked eye during brain surgery: a dull, yellowish rim around the opalescent white brain. Gliosis protects the surrounding brain from injury, but only for a while. In time, it may become the origin for aberrant incoherent electricity – seizures. So, at a biological level your immediate response to trauma is protective but, over time, it gets in the way. At a behavioural level, the same thing can happen. The trauma can return in overwhelming ways, the aftershocks

upending and intruding on the patient's world, causing depression, profound anxiety, or some uniquely
personal and painful combination causing Post Traumatic Stress Disorder (PTSD).

PTSD is not based on a blood test or some other
objective measure but on a set of observations; it's a
shorthand for the specific misery some people experience in the aftermath of trauma. The abbreviation has
become part of the popular lexicon, watered down,
simplified, trivialized to describe our reactions to the
hassles and discomforts of everyday life. What the
diagnosis sets out to describe, however, is anything
but trivial. It is characterized by three sets of persistent symptoms: re-experiencing the trauma through
flashbacks and nightmares; avoiding emotional attachments; and hyperarousal, which can cause sufferers
to startle easily, to feel on edge and anger quickly.
Common perceptions of which gender or type of
person is prone to PTSD don't tell a nuanced story. For
example, some soldiers experience PTSD without
ever going into combat, and after sexual trauma, men
have a higher incidence of PTSD than women.

For most people suffering from trauma, their symptoms don't conform to a tidy checklist; they defy easy
classification. But their suffering is no less real for
that. By definition, PTSD requires physical trauma,
but emotional trauma can cause the same devastating
symptoms as physical trauma and bring the same
unbidden vigilance and intrusive memories.

With so much coming at us, our brains are built to forget far more than we remember. They have evolved to understand the world in broad brushstrokes, not to remember each pixel from the past. Forgetting most of the flotsam and jetsam of everyday life – a phone number or where you parked the car yesterday – helps us remember what's important. It's called adaptive forgetting. Most memories fade, like an old photograph, losing their emotional punch, along with many of the details, but memories of a trauma can last, and mental images of a trauma can reappear, unwanted – the attacker's plaid shirt or the red car just before it hits you. Trauma can make us fearful of the people, places and objects that were present when it occurred.

Memories are initially fragile, like sculptures made of soft clay that have yet to set. We can pick up new information – a wifi password, say – right away, but to commit something to memory requires time. Our brains need to consolidate the information in the far-reaching assembly of neurons that make memory meaningful enough to really hold on to. Emotion is the shortcut to consolidation, taking away the usually requisite time and repetition to imprint a memory deeply. Memories aren't saved in a single spot like a file on a hard drive. A memory is more of a web, and it is stored in different regions of the brain.

Emotional memories are consolidated in the brain within hours. Once memories are set, once that brief window has closed, those memories are much more resistant to change. That means what you do during that time immediately after a traumatic event is crucial. It seems that what we're doing just after we experience trauma, before the memory is consolidated, has a profound impact on how the trauma affects us – and whether it can continue to reach into our present to traumatize us anew. During the French Revolution, *les tricoteuses* famously sat by the guillotine, knitting; apparently, they suffered no post-traumatic stress. Somehow, the task of knitting seems to have protected them.

British psychologist Emily Holmes believes visual spatial tasks such as knitting may prevent traumatic memories from sticking in the mind. She found that playing the game *Tetris* before memories consolidated helps block flashbacks of traumatic events. Likewise, participants who tapped out a specific pattern on a hidden keyboard while they watched videos showing the bloody aftermath of real car accidents suffered fewer intrusive memories than those who didn't perform the task. Those performing a verbal task while they watched the gruesome videos – counting by threes – had more intrusive memories.

Darwin suggested that inappropriately prolonged escape or avoidance behaviour would put an animal at a disadvantage. Avoidance also puts us at a disadvantage when it comes to traumatic memories. Under the right conditions, recalling traumatic events may heal the emotional injury of a trauma and lead to 'fear extinction' through a process called reconsolidation. Creating a memory is not a one-time procedure, forever unchanging, like a sculpture chiselled in granite. A memory is malleable. If a memory is retrieved, it needs to be reconsolidated, re-remembered. This is a biological process: protein synthesis makes the memory vulnerable to change and provides an opportunity. New information and new context can be added to the original memory.

Remarkably, some trauma turns to growth – a reverse PTSD. Post-traumatic growth is positive psychological change resulting from struggle. It might mean a new appreciation of life, an openness to possibilities, a reordering of priorities. Despite the trauma, personal growth is possible in its aftermath, but only for those willing to put in work to make sense of the world turned upside down, to reframe the event and reconsolidate the memory.

Some patients diagnosed with cancer who feel stressed and anxious soon after the diagnosis are able to achieve post-traumatic growth over time. The initial struggle is instrumental in the ultimate growth. Stroke patients and adolescent tornado survivors who reflect on what happened and worked to make sense of it, positively reconstructing the event in their minds, were more likely to achieve post-traumatic growth. This act of positive reflection is called deliberate rumination.

Strangely, those who experience more psychological disruption have the potential to experience more growth than those who are armed with greater resilience. This transformational coping doesn't mean a reduction in pain or an increase in feelings of well-being but instead a level of functioning that is higher than before the trauma. Those who are better at dealing with adversity may not achieve the same post-traumatic growth because their perception of the event does not reach the critical level of seismicity. They aren't rattled enough for the event to trigger growth in them.

Difficult times hold the deepest reservoir from which to draw post-traumatic growth. This counter-intuitive, trauma-induced flourishing can come about in a number of ways, all of them leading back to the subjective experience of the trauma itself. Those able to thrive after trauma demonstrate an ability to reframe or recast the trauma. In interviews with survivors of major trauma, an acceptance of the turn of events was a recurring observation, regardless of the nature of the event. 'You don't choose the issues that you've got, but you can – you can – make a choice to change,' one person said. Another told the researchers something I've heard many times: 'I am who I am because of what happened.'

One of my patients was a chronic worrier before his cancer diagnosis. To his family's surprise, the diagnosis put an end to his constant fretting. He said he no longer had time to waste on it, since his time was limited. Another patient responded to advanced breast cancer with a ferocious drive to keep working between visits and therapies. She was a bus driver, and she said it offered the perfect balance between thinking about cancer and forgetting about cancer. Faced with the trauma of a cancer diagnosis, each made sense of their new world and thrived in their own ways.

When we pull on the web of our memories, our mind unspools sights, smells and emotions connected to that web. That day after the motorway pile-up, the clothes on the floor reminded me of those plane-crash victims whose clothes were settling like leaves. This memory had been undisturbed and unremembered for fifteen years. Like a spark, I also remembered the sharp smell of burning flesh under the blazing jet fuel at the scene; unrecognized then, now a smell I'm accustomed to from surgery. We can't control when memories emerge or how they will affect us. I was lucky. When those vivid memories of the plane crash returned, I had a professional relationship with trauma, allowing me to frame it in a less psychologically jarring context. It might have been more traumatic if I'd chosen a different line of work.

While most people avoid trauma, some surgeons seek it out. I certainly did. As trainees in the general trauma service, we were looking for action. When a patient is really on the brink, the surgeon's pager reads 'trauma resus' (short for 'trauma resuscitation') and patient and surgeon are brought straight into the operating theatre.

With the passing of laws requiring seat belts everything changed for trauma surgeons. The patient rarely needed to be rushed to the operating theatre for emergency surgery. Infrequently did they need exploratory laparotomies, or 'ex-laps', where a patient's belly is opened with huge vertical incisions, the kind used by coroners during autopsies. Hundreds of young surgeons understood what the change meant. Those who went into surgery not for the money but for the gore and the glory, the prestige and the competition, knew their licence had largely been revoked to participate in something so exhilarating and so unnatural: delivering trauma to heal.

Over the years, emergency surgery and its heroics became less common. When handing patients over to the next shift, we would bemoan the lack of emergency surgeries after the long day and night of work. The tally might be twelve resuses, none operative, ten in the ICU and two on the general ward. When we signed out at the end of shifts, 'none operative' was the salient detail, offered up in disappointed tones. Don't get me wrong. We didn't want people to get hurt. We just coveted the opportunity to use our hands and our skills to rescue those whose fates we didn't create.

On the general trauma team, it was usually a fully-fledged surgeon who made the call for belly or chest trauma surgery. Legs and arms were wrapped with cardboard and had to wait. It was different for neurosurgery. Neurosurgeons were so rare that most nights we didn't have a single fully trained brain surgeon in the hospital. Because of the scarcity of neurosurgeons, ours was the only discipline where a mere trainee who was 'in house' could make the call to 'take someone back' – take someone to the operating room for surgery.

The decision whether or not one's skull should be opened fell solely upon the brain-surgery trainee – and not an experienced trainee at that – a second-year (out of seven) trainee. Even calling it 'second year' is a stretch because the first year is the internship year, and you rarely operate during it. So, essentially, a novice surgeon, a rookie. Thirteen months out of medical school where you observe but do little. Go ahead and make the call on essentially your first month of being a 'brain surgeon': whether this type of brain injury warrants a frantic rush through the hallways to the operating theatre. It was a thrill because of the possibility for heroics, but with it came angst and fear and worry over whether cutting this person open was justified. The first time I made that call, I was twenty-seven, and the responsibility was exhilarating. That moment and concept is so much bigger than Hollywood tales of 'stopping a bleeder'. A podiatrist can stop a bleeder. By deciding to send someone back or not, I was deciding their fate. A correct decision meant opening the patient's skull. A wrong call could worsen their traumatic injury.

I hadn't even taken out an appendix, and I was making the solo call to take a patient back to brain surgery while an experienced neurosurgeon drove in. Before medical images could be shared on cell-phones and computers, those on call at home relied entirely on the assessment of the brain surgeons in training. A room on the operating floor is always saved for trauma resuses, and I called out to the trauma bay – to the anaesthesiologists, the professors of trauma surgery, the senior nurses around me. I said two simple words with engineered poise. They knew I knew little, but they also knew the structure: brain-surgery trainees make calls that only senior surgeons made in other specialties. The two words were 'trauma craniotomy', which meant I had to open the skull as quickly as possible.

I made a judgement call that the cap had to come off this fizzing bottle. When I was training in general surgery, I'd watched veteran neurosurgeons do it and now I was the one making the call. Does this patient really need this surgery, or can they be kept under observation a while longer? I made that call. Then, still dealing with the aftershocks of doubt, I had to steer my thoughts to the dangerous work ahead. I didn't want to make a mistake while waiting for back-up – before a senior surgeon arrived to fix and finish.

And then I heard the door smash open and the professor backed in with sopping scrubbed hands, ready to take over. And he said the words that made this not a calamity: 'He needed to go – I would have made the same call.' At the time, I wasn't even thinking about who this human was. I was thinking about myself. My feelings. My fear of faltering. My potential trauma. I don't remember anything else about that patient. Patient X. Just a moment. A burden. A responsibility. An opportunity.

In your lifetime, it's likely you'll have to deal with a traumatic event – it may be long and slow; it may be fast and unexpected. In the moment the trauma arrives, step one is to survive – simply survive. And for that there is no script; in that crisis, whatever one can draw upon is of value. But the ripples of trauma endured are incessant, and we must revisit the trauma on our own terms and on our own timeline, never letting it sit seemingly idle. Unless we tend to it, it will become psychologically corrosive. Struggling with trauma is not a sign of failure but the necessary groundwork for personal growth.

Traumatic energy won't just pass through us; it must be metabolized. It is a catalyst for an aftermath you didn't want but now are responsible for directing. What I didn't know that day in the trauma bay was that decades of caring for those dealing with trauma would also fortify me. I learned from my patients' adversity, without having to bear the real weight. Their life lessons would guide me through my challenges. Unimaginable are the complexities I would have missed if it were not for my experience with trauma at such an early point in my life.

2.

Performance

He came to me, a nineteen-year-old with a time bomb in his head. Scheduled as the seventh patient in my Friday clinic, he brought notes from the two neuro-surgeons who had already seen him. An artery in his brain was dangerously malformed and at risk of exploding due to an aneurysm, a spot where the blood vessel is stretched thin and, like a balloon, in danger of bursting. With each heartbeat, a pressure wave rippled out from his heart and risked tearing the artery. With each heartbeat, he was gripped with fear. His name was Richard.

If the vessel ruptured, his heart would send a puls-ing cascade of blood into the skull, irritating the surface of the brain and damaging its cells. At the same time, the part of his brain the artery was sup-posed to supply with oxygen-rich blood would be starved. A rupture carries a 40 per cent chance of death, so no surprise that he was terrified.

The good news is that surgery for these cases usu-ally goes smoothly. I explained to Richard that the risk of leaving the aneurysm untreated was higher than the risk of surgery: both could cause devastating brain injury to his language function or death. This is heavy news at any age but unimaginably intense for someone just beginning their adult life. Richard chose to have me perform the surgery in June, giving him the summer to recuperate.

The operation he needed is established in surgical lore for being technically challenging; most neurosurgeons won't even take it on. It has the most extreme range of outcomes: on one end the patient is cured; on the other, the patient dies.

When I perform any surgery, not only the difficult cases, I stick to a ritual. Eliminating extraneous variables allows me to focus. The ritual has been refined over the years to give me the best chance to excel. During the surgery I'll be standing and leaning in awkward positions throughout the day, so the night before, I go to the gym. No hard lifting, just light work before I go into battle the next day.

The patients arrive at 5 a.m., well before sunrise, for a 7.30 a.m. surgery. The nurses come in at around 6.45 a.m. to get the room set up. Surgeons and anaesthesiologists turn up at seven. I park in my usual spot; it's not reserved for me, but at that hour it's rarely taken.

I walk to the area where my patients usually wait, Station 6. Richard had been checked in, changed into a hospital gown that ties at the back, and had an IV put in one arm. It must be unnerving for patients to see so many strangers before that big moment, a surgery that could well determine how their lives from that point play out. I like to think that the sight of others who have signed up for something crazy – to be cut open – reassures them that they are in a safe space, despite it being stuffed to the brim with tools that would look horrific in any other context.

In the locker room I change into fresh scrubs: alongside people with two-year technical degrees, college degrees, medical degrees, and people who have never been to university. When I was a medical student, the tattoo on my right forearm often led me to be confused for a member of the 'turnover' crew – the caretakers who mop up the blood from the floors and machines before the instruments for the next case can be brought into the operating theatre. I never minded as long I could get my chance centre stage to help the patients having surgery.

Before entering the operating theatre, across a thick red line, you have to don a hairnet and then wash your hands and forearms. The patient is on a ventilator. The final step in the pre-surgery ritual is the 'timeout'; all hospitals in the US must do this before we can start making the incision. The timeout is run by a nurse and we all have to stand still for ten seconds while the patient's name is read out, along with the terms of consent and the name of the planned operation. Then the anaesthesiologist, surgeon and surgical nurse must all say, 'Agree.' It's like the safety check when you sit in the emergency aisle on an aeroplane. Only when everyone has uttered their audible consent can surgery begin.

For this operation on Richard, in particular, everything had to be done in a rhythm; unnecessary urgency leads to mistakes. I shaved his head and doused it with an orange sterilizing liquid called Betadine. A technician placed electrodes on his head to monitor brainwaves, another safety net. The anaesthesiologist had ample blood in the room. Now it was my turn. The clock read 8.15.

The aneurysm was in the middle cerebral artery, a deep and vital vessel which divides into dozens of offshoots as it moves towards the top of the brain's canopy. To find the middle cerebral artery I had to separate the frontal lobe from the temporal lobe by opening the Sylvian fissure that holds them together. This treacherous valley was my planned pathway to the target artery. I parted the iridescent membranes and slid between the brain lobes, ensuring no violation to the brain tissue. The clock now read 9.15.

The wall of the aneurysmal dome was thin enough for the whorls of blood flowing with each heartbeat to be visible. My own heart beat fast, but my elevated heart rate wasn't a sign of anxiety or panic. I was calm. My focus was unfettered. Being cool under pressure doesn't mean your body hasn't responded to the situation, that you're somehow immune to the circumstances. I knew the stakes. Having a fast heart rate is part of the exhilaration in a situation like this.

The key and critical manoeuvre is to place a small spring-loaded titanium clip at the base of the aneurysm. All this happens so deep inside the skull that only one person – the surgeon – can work. With the titanium clip at the tip of my eight-inch forceps, I was now ready to squeeze it into position with my trigger finger and thumb and deliver it to the target. The clip prevents blood from flowing into the aneurysm, eliminating the risk of it bursting. Until it was in place, the aneurysm posed an existential threat to the patient. I moved slowly, gently releasing the jaws of the clip around the base of the bulge ballooning from the blood vessel. The clip was almost closed around the base when the aneurysm exploded. The artery violently sprayed blood from the tear. Torrential bleeding welled out of the patient's skull. The clock read 9.45.

No simulated crash landing can fully prepare you. No imagining of a crisis can truly ready you. It's not just about knowing what the manoeuvres are; the hardest part is being steady enough to pull them off. The gushing blood obscured what I could see. The low blood pressure alert caught the anaesthesiologist's attention. I looked at her and said: *give blood*. While other organs can last for hours without blood, the brain needs to be irrigated so desperately even minutes of drought wilt its tissue, causing a stroke.

When we're under pressure and our actions have

real consequences, it's easy to become overwhelmed. In 1979, during the partial core meltdown at the Three Mile Island nuclear power plant in Pennsylvania, operators were disoriented by all the alarms. Facing the threat of catastrophe, they didn't know which alarms were the most pressing and which could be ignored. There is a name for this: alarm overload. More alarms are received than can be addressed. Under pressure to perform, our brains, too, can become over-whelmed by a surfeit of signals. To respond quickly and effectively in a crisis, we need a way to bring order to the external alarms, to find focus by ignoring emo-tional distractors. Evolution has supplied us with a way to do just that.

For a long time, the basal ganglia were thought to be associated solely with the control of movement. Now, this paired cluster of neurons in the emotional brain has been shown to be involved in sensory con-trol as well as something that has been dubbed 'active interference'. Instead of shining a spotlight on what is important, our brains actively filter out what is deemed unimportant. When you are being inundated with stimuli, the basal ganglia filter what should be let through.

Devoting too much attention to the irrelevant would exhaust your fuel supply, because the brain is such an energy glutton. It makes up only 2 per cent of body weight but demands 20 per cent of your energy. Neural efficiency matters. Oddly, perhaps, neural activity is lower in experts, whether it's professional rifle shooters or memory champions. They don't dial up the focus, they dial down the distraction and stress. This neural efficiency is the real talent of experts under pressure. The ability to be vigilant is not an achievement; it is built in. The ability to ignore, however, must be cultivated.

I'd never seen a ruptured aneurysm, but I knew what I could do. Now, I needed to place several clamps to rebuild the torn wall of the artery. Each time I tried, I failed. Six attempts at various manoeuvres got me nowhere. The clock read 10.45. I persisted, but failed again and again. The clock now read 11.50.

The patient had received fifteen pints and the empty blood bags lay on the floor. At this point, all his own blood had escaped, replaced by that of strangers. In over two hours, I'd made no progress. My mind was definitely full, too full, almost seeping out of my skull with the weight of what was upon me. Opening the dam was the only way to repair the dam. Let the deluge run too long, and the blood volume would drop to a point where the heart failed. So, in between my attempts to repair the torn artery, I'd pause. Then the anaesthesiologist would try to replenish the blood volume, which we call 'tanking up', before I tried once again to complete the necessary manoeuvre.

In those gaps of time when the anaesthesiologist was tanking up the patient after every failed effort, my own brain struggled to keep surging adrenaline in its place. I could feel those chemicals being released from my reptilian brain, signalling danger, activating rapid breathing, redirecting blood flow. Panic was creeping in at the edges and needed to be held at bay. This internal conflict – thought versus emotion – was running through me and I had to find the balance that would let me perform the operation effectively. Most surgeons don't go into surgery where the stakes are extremely high. Most surgeries aren't life-threatening. This one was about to be. These manoeuvres can only be performed several times; then your window closes and there is the possibility you will be facing the thing that strikes terror in surgeons – intraoperative death, the patient going cold on the operating table. What would I say to his family? Who could I call to help? But I knew these were false passages. These distracting thoughts were competing with and exhausting my attention. Remember: focus is not about heightened attention, it's about better suppression of distraction. The prefrontal cortex, where this is all processed, would be overwhelmed with inputs if we weren't able to filter out distractions. But that filter easily becomes porous when emotion is added to the mix.

When the patient was being given another transfusion, I had a few minutes, a small window, before I had to get back to repairing the dam under high flow. My forceps held a piece of dense cloth – a patty – to prevent the brisk egress of blood from a critical vessel ten inches deep in Richard's skull. With the bleeding temporarily stemmed, and while more blood was being squeezed in, I used the time to steady my breathing. In situations like this, I don't breathe more deeply, I breathe more slowly. Three seconds in; three seconds out. No sudden inhalation of panic, and no quick dumping of air with mouth agape. I find it's easier to pace my breathing by inhaling and exhaling through my nose.

With this measured breathing, I am taking advantage of human physiology. Meditative breathing can moderate the electrical activity in our brain. This has been proven by research done on patients with epilepsy. Electrodes were surgically inserted under the skull and on to the surface of the brains in order to locate the epicentre of the seizures. In hospital for a period of time, a group of patients participated in various thinking experiments, one of which was meditative breathing. Direct intracranial measurements demonstrated that breathing patterns, by changing the electricity in the brain, can steer it towards anxiety or towards calm.

Meditative breathing keeps us from slipping into an adaptive state that served us well in the distant past when we had to run from immediate threat – hyperventilation. Danger and breathing are intimately linked. When we sense looming danger, the brain sends signals and readies the lungs and diaphragm. When you flee from a threat, your muscles go into a higher gear, and the muscle cells churn out metabolic waste, the most critical of which is a gas – carbon dioxide.

We hyperventilate when we're facing danger in order to speed up the gas exchange in our lungs. If your muscles are not pumping but your brain is still sending signals to breathe faster, you are blowing off too much carbon dioxide and this can leave an inadequate amount in your blood. This creates problems of its own, especially if you're in the middle of surgery with a young man's life at stake. Hyperventilation exacerbates fright and leaves you jittery, twitchy, off your game – just when you need to be focused. That is why controlling your breathing is step one of crisis management.

Learning to control your breathing is the most powerful weapon you have to strengthen your emotional regulation and, in turn, improve your performance. It's better not to wait for the moment of crisis to turn to this safety valve. When it's a daily habit, it's easier to deploy it effectively when you need it.

Early in my training, I noticed that experienced surgeons used a strip of tape to seal their surgical mask to the bridge of their nose and put one on either cheek, just below the eyes. In brain surgery, you wear surgical loupes, glasses with jeweller's lenses that give 3x magnification, and the tape prevents these fogging up, especially when, under pressure to perform, your breathing becomes fast and heavy. I used to do this too, but now I don't. When my field of view fogs from my breath, that tells me I'm doing something wrong, and so I control my breath, its rate and its depth. Get that cadence right or performance will suffer, as will the patient.

Standing over Richard, my breathing again under my control, my thinking cleared. I was down to my last option, my final manoeuvre. I asked the anaesthesiologist to administer adenosine, a drug that would temporarily stop Richard's heart beating, flat-lining him but also creating a zero-blood-flow state so that I could properly see the base of the spewing arterial bubble where the clip needed to be applied. On the monitor to my left, a readout from the electrodes on Richard's scalp showed his dancing brainwaves. On the monitor to my right, the reading of the EKG electrodes on his chest indicated his heart rhythm. That moment when Richard's heart was no longer beating but his brain was not yet starved of blood was the loneliest place I'd ever been. But it did give me one shot, one clear view to repair the aneurysm. I prepared and placed three clips in a quick sequence to reconstitute the vessel wall. I watched as the blood surged back through the vessel. Fortunately, it held. The heart was chemically restarted and Richard's brainwaves never stopped dancing.

The clock read 12.50.

Some surgeries pose incredible technical challenges, putting the skills of even the best surgeon to the ultimate test. Other times, unprecedented and unforeseen crises arise, rearing up like aliens, throwing up a level of complexity that you won't find in any textbook and which you wouldn't see again if you performed the surgery a thousand more times. These rare cases require crisis management in the way Houdini performed crisis management, locked in a straitjacket and dumped in a tank of water. The clock is ticking, and the surgeon needs to act with clarity, precision and skill. And, all the while, the stakes could not be higher. In such situations, it is vital to hold back the creeping edges of panic that will erode your ability to make the most effective decisions and to deploy the most effective tactics.

After surgery, Richard was kept asleep on machines in the ICU to give his brain time to heal; there is inevitably swelling after such invasive brain surgery. When I gradually woke him up after a week, he was fine, both physically and mentally. And grateful that he was all there. He took a few months off to regain his full strength and then went back to college.

These days, patients with the deadliest diseases seek me out. I'm grateful for this: it's how I make a difference to the world, using my skills to change lives in a way that others won't or can't do. It may seem strange, but I don't dread these moments. It's where I give my best. It's when I'm at my best. True performance is always performance under pressure, when the result really matters. Good hands are not enough – you need nerve.

The legendary early-twentieth-century neurosurgeon Harvey Cushing, known as a hard-driving but brilliant teacher, put it this way: 'The capacity of man himself is only revealed when, under stress and responsibility, he breaks through his educational shell, and he may then be a splendid surprise to himself no less than to his teachers.'

Great performers are not immune to pressure; they have simply learned to manage it. Preparation is key. Visualization can be helpful. Mental practice of a physical activity can enhance performance. If you've ever used various methods to calm your nerves before an interview or to get psyched up before a big performance, you're probably already familiar with mental preparation. But mental practice is a particular technique that entails sitting quietly and imagining yourself performing the task from start to finish. Rehearsing in your mind works because you're activating many of the same neurons as you would if you were actually doing it. Imagine playing a Bach sonata note for note, and you are activating the same parts of your brain as if you were really playing the piano.

For me, it's important not only to visualize what I want to do but to create crisis scenarios in my mind to visualize my response when it all goes south. I imagine disruptions to the plan in a complicated case before I fall asleep: If this happens, then what are my manoeuvres? Around this corner, what could there be? I have always found imagining the challenge ahead and the various ways it could go worthwhile. Remarkably, the electricity of our thoughts can be detected before we actually register having the thought. Rituals may help get you focused and check-lists are helpful but, ultimately, it is only when we are faced with a real crisis that our ability to perform under pressure is truly revealed.

What actually happens when the unimaginable forces you to make decisions in the moment? Captain Chesley 'Sully' Sullenberger pulled off an emergency landing on the Hudson River when both engines of the packed passenger jet he was flying lost power following a bird strike over New York City in 2009. How? What is shared by brains that excel under pressure? And what can we learn from their exceptional performance that we might harness and apply? To answer that, anatomy and biology are not enough. We need to peer at the brain's electrical physiology.

In Portuguese-born writer Fernando Pessoa's *Book of Disquiet*, published half a century after his death in 1935, he mused: 'I do not know what instruments, what violins and harps, drums and tambours sound and clash inside me. I know myself only as a symphony.' Now, we do know. Pessoa's inner symphony is the communication between neurons, electrochemical signals that form the basis of all thought, emotion and behaviour. It is an orchestra of staggering complexity.

When neurons spark in concert, like an orchestra, the electrical activity coalesces into brainwaves, oscillations that can be measured by the amplitude and frequency of their collective discharge and then categorized. The brain has five different types of brainwave, but when they are part of an ensemble, their output is infinite. One hertz (Hz) equals a frequency of one cycle per second. Brainwaves range from .5 Hz to up to 35 Hz. Delta waves are the slowest, and occur when you are in a deep, dreamless sleep. Theta waves come next, experienced while daydreaming or deep in meditation. Alpha waves are in the middle, between 8 Hz and 12 Hz, produced when you are relaxed and not focused on anything. Beta waves are the second fastest, coming when you are awake and alert. Gamma waves are the quickest, pulsing around 30 Hz, when your brain is processing information and learning.

It is possible to detect the 'hidden orchestra' from outside the skull, like recording a roar from outside a stadium, with an electroencephalogram, or EEG. It's a powerful tool, but it doesn't say much about the orchestra's constituents or components. However, in another way, it tells us more than the individual components ever could: it reveals what they achieve together.

The alpha-wave rhythm is also known as the Berger

wave, after German psychiatrist Hans Berger. In 1924, he attached electrodes near the scars of a teenager who had a hole in his skull after undergoing surgery to remove a tumour. He connected them to a galvanometer, which translates brain activity into wavy lines on photographic paper. And so the EEG was born. Even with the advent of new imaging technology such as MRI and CT scans, the electro-encephalogram still has a key part to play: it detects global energy phenomena about the brain's electro-physiology that tells a unique story of our minds that brain scans cannot.

Talking about energy and electricity with regard to the brain may sound like something you wouldn't hear from a biologist, but it's actually a fairly accurate description. Our brains have been known to be electric since the Romans treated migraines with jolts of electricity from the black torpedo fish, an electric ray. Our brains are so electric the composite charge could switch on a light bulb, but to consider our brains turning on and off like a light bulb gives the wrong impression. The signals in our brain are defined by tone, modulation and drift. Thinking is not a light bulb going on but a flow of electrical energy more akin to the beautiful loops and whorls of a school of fish, or a flock of starlings in flight, their murmuration almost rolling backwards and tumbling over itself. To consider the individual fish or bird is to miss everything. Thought is so much more than an individual neuron firing. One neuron is a desert. Two neurons allow electricity to flow. One hundred billion do something indescribable. That's what brainwaves are – currents, tidal movements that happen under the seemingly placid ocean surface. That is consciousness. That is our mind. That is us.

When you're completely absorbed in an activity, you're said to be in a flow state. You lose track of time, of your surroundings. You are not subject to life's many distractions, or even to your own sense of self or self-consciousness. And in the flow state, our performance flourishes. Mihaly Csikszentmihalyi proposed the concept of flow, describing it as the 'holistic sensation that people feel when they act with total involvement'. In *Beyond Boredom and Anxiety*, he wrote that flow represents peak enjoyment, energetic focus and creative concentration. When we are in a flow state, we temporarily distance ourselves from our own prefrontal cortex and one of its many roles – task-oriented behaviour. We're in a state of neural efficiency, less thought and less emotion, which allows us to become absorbed in what we're doing.

Our brains produce alpha waves when we are in a state of wakeful rest. The brain is not engaged in a specific task, it's more like an idling engine, in neutral. You experience alpha waves just after waking up, or when you are not thinking of anything in particular. Alpha waves are associated with creativity, with ideas and inspiration.

In some operations, there are moments when you can feel out of control; it's a bit like being in free fall. There's a threat, but you still have time to act. The manoeuvres I try are not typed up on a laminated checklist. I'm not a machine, and neither is the patient. Flesh and disease meld in myriad ways in cancer. Pulling a patient out of a difficult moment takes improvisation. It takes alpha waves and creativity, formed in response to the unique set of conditions presented, and the manoeuvres you try on different cases are like branches with positive turns, negative turns and, sometimes, dead ends. It's like those 'choose your own adventure' books. Your choices and how you respond to the various obstacles determine not just if the patient lives but how damaged they will be as a result of the tally of missteps. Sometimes you see the missteps only in the rear-view mirror.

Describing flow, Csikszentmihalyi wrote, 'The best moments usually occur when a person's body or mind is stretched to its limits in a voluntary effort to accomplish something difficult and worthwhile.' For me, personally, I would add risk. Somewhere between the benign fright of a scary movie and the real terror of being attacked exists a space I love, a thrill that calls upon a different side of me.

Embracing a challenge that requires holding intrusive thoughts at bay and releasing focus can force you to step outside time into a state of calm. For me, this can happen in surgery. When you are performing at your highest level, it's like turning a cacophony into a symphony. You are achieving flow, but flow itself is not the goal. Flow is not a solution unto itself, but you can use its advantages to create the mindset needed in order to handle crises. Flow is the elixir for coming through in the clutch, under pressure. These moments are a deeply meditative state for me, but there is more to it.

For me, flow in surgery has an element of rapture. When I'm in that space, in that energy, the same chemicals, growth factors and hormones are at play. Only high stakes can give you this unique and rare experience. This is followed immediately by relief when a dangerous manoeuvre is successfully completed, and then a calm that can only be experienced after the eruption of all the ammunition, all the brain chemicals – a deep calm, a euphoria of sorts. The energy is all-encompassing. For years, finding these cases where I could perform at my absolute best was a need that drove me.

3.

Self

As I walked up to the patient in the ICU, his eyes directed my gaze to the lower half of the bed. The two corners were perfectly tucked in and the bedding was taut. It looked like a hotel bed that hadn't been slept in. Even though I'd known what to expect, the sight caught me off guard. As my gaze moved back up the bed, the man's form picked up halfway, his ribcage rising and falling under the hospital sheet. He looked like a living CPR mannequin, a torso and head and nothing else.

The patient had undergone a surgery called a hemicorpectomy. His body below the waist had been amputated. I was the surgeon who dealt the final blow after other teams of surgeons sawed through and removed his sacrum, genitals and legs.

The ICU is shaped like a horseshoe, not unlike Los Angeles International Airport, with its terminals on the outer perimeter. A wise nurse had placed the man in the end slot, with the least traffic. It was the day after surgery and his face showed pain, despite the heavy drip of morphine meant to assuage both emotional and physical suffering. His expression was sullen and the corners of his mouth lacked any upward turn, something I often see in patients on heavy IV narcotics.

I took in the hospital bed and what was left of the person in it. Who we are, our notion of self, is a combination of body, mind and the autobiographical narrative we create for ourselves. As my eyes returned to his, I wondered if he was the same person he had been when I'd first seen him. I wondered if I was. We didn't say anything to each other.

I'd come in late. I'd wanted to drop my sons off at school, and since I hadn't received a call, I figured no crisis had occurred. He had already seen a parade of doctors that morning. I decided to wait to talk with him the next day, when the meds had been tapered and we had both had some time to process what had happened to him – and my role in it.

The plan made sense, in theory. Cut out the cancer, all of it, and you can improve the chance of the patient living. We cut off limbs to cure cancer, so why not both limbs and the pelvis? This brute-force approach has been around for more than a century, ever since influential London surgeon W. Sampson Handley advanced what he called 'the theory of centrifugal lymphatic permeation', which argued that cancer spreads from its point of origin and so surgery can potentially remove the cancer and cure the patient. Before that, physicians tended to follow the teachings of Hippocrates and Galen, who thought cancer was incurable.

Taking Handley's theory to heart, American professor of surgery William Stewart Halsted developed a radical operation for breast cancer, making a large incision, removing the mammary gland, both pectoral muscles and nearby lymph nodes. The radical mastectomy did improve the odds of the patient surviving, though little thought was given to their quality of life afterwards. The surgery is now rarely performed.

Still, the impulse to go after the cancer is always there. To cut it out: to remove it by any means necessary. This isn't only true for surgeons but for patients, too. I've had patients plead, 'Can you please get it out of me?', even when I've told them it won't do anything for their chances. They want to be liberated. They are asking for a de-alienation, a rehumanization.

Usually, when I perform surgery, my approach is the result of a conversation between the patient and me. Every patient is different. In clinic, surgeons have a limited allotment of time to connect with patients and decide what to do. Patients read energy. If you can't connect in the first few minutes, it won't happen.

I tell my patients, 'You are driving your life, and I want to show you some images of what's happening inside you – why you might be struggling with pain or disability.' I take time to make it clear that, 'This is you,' while I point to their name and birthdate on an image on a twenty-five-inch monitor. I want them to know this isn't some stock photo. This is your body and this is your cancer. It's part of my approach to personalized medicine. I'll show a patient the tumour and tell them that this ball of tissue doesn't follow your rules. The cancer has defied the biological programming designed to shut it down and declared its independence. It has its own nefarious identity, its own liberated self.

Then, I invite their response. Some are fighting for every month. Others are looking for a gracious exit. Some opt for one of the smaller operations in my arsenal. Some never come back. Some sign up for surgery and are thankful. Some have regret for choosing too much surgery. I am at their crossroads with them, but every patient understands that they are driving. I'm informing and explaining, but they are behind the wheel, navigating their lives despite the tremendous fear and uncertainty of a cancer diagnosis. It's a heroic display of resilience.

With the man undergoing a hemicorpectomy, his cancer was in the pelvis and the decision to remove the lower half of his body wasn't something the two of us had decided. The plan was the result of collaboration between a team of doctors with different specialties, members of the hospital's Tumour Board. The multidisciplinary team came up with an aggressive sequence of operations to rid him of his cancer. The plan was a long shot, a Hail Mary, really: cut it out, radiate it and then chemo it. This last step was the equivalent of spraying the lawn with herbicide after you've pulled out the weeds, the goal to kill any seeds that remained. The seeds, in this analogy, are cancer cells.

I said nothing at the Tumour Board meeting as the team conceived this approach but with my silence I'd agreed to be a participant, I was complicit. My part wasn't technically challenging, and I acquiesced. I was trying to respect the patient's wishes. But neither the patient nor I realized at the time that cutting off his bottom half would be too much.

It's a weird thing when you can dangle the word 'cure' into the conversation, even when it's done fairly. Even if there's a 10 per cent chance, the patient hears nothing other than that there is a chance of winning, and they certainly don't calculate what it costs to get that winning lottery ticket. When they have that glimmer of hope in their eyes, the patient struggles to see anything but the chance of surviving. Despite the harrowing odds, even the narrowest percentage gives them a shot. Most advanced cancers and brain cancers don't have even the smallest chance of having that opportunity. They cannot be cured. The cancer has spread, metastasized. With surgery, patients are merely looking to buy time, to beat back the invader. Because this patient's cancer had not spread, he had a rare opportunity. He had a chance to be cured of his cancer with surgery. The cost was what surgeons call 'a wide margin', removing tissue some distance from the tumour to ensure that all the cancer cells have been excised.

When I saw the patient before surgery, he was getting around on his own, using a walker because of the pain from his hip. He was enthusiastic about the operation, experiencing a cognitive dissonance: a 10 per cent chance of a cure means a 90 per cent chance of no cure but, as with most patients, he saw only that 10 per cent. Also, calling the operation he was about to undergo 'radical' is an understatement. With a hemicorpectomy, more of the body is missing post-operatively than with any other surgery. There is no prosthesis that can replace the lower half of your body; the only possibility is a bucket seat so the patient can sit upright. How can someone possibly be expected to give informed consent for something so drastic? The idea is to extend life, but at what cost? Neither the patient nor the physicians on the multi-disciplinary team spent much time talking about this patient's quality of life following surgery.

The whole process was a strange thrill for this patient: a team of four doctors had seen him and were focused on helping him 'beat' cancer. He was detailing his journey on social media, but the day after surgery he stopped posting and fell off the grid.

The American surgeon Frederick Kredel first proposed the hemicorpectomy in 1950 for locally advanced cancer limited to the pelvis – cases just like that of this patient. Kredel had a different name for the procedure: a 'halfectomy'. The first attempt was a decade later, and the procedure remains rare and risky, at the unmarked border of surgical heroism and hubris.

During the surgery, the abdominal surgeons lassoed the end of the man's bowels and pulled the last funnel out to a hole in the skin near his belly button. A plastic tube was inserted to drain urine from his kidneys, and his reproductive organs were cut out. The next part is where I came in. It was my job to cut the patient's spinal column in half. To fully disconnect the bottom half of the man's body, his spine and the delicate glistening tail of the brain, the spinal cord, nestled inside it, would need to be dissected, divided and tied off. Although, technically, it was simple, this is the most important part of the surgery. Tying off the spinal cord prevents the brain fluid the spinal cord bathes in – the same brain fluid that is made by the brain itself – from pouring out, and the moment the spinal cord is divided, the man would be forever separated from himself.

The surgery was deemed a success. The cancer was excised, along with the lower half of the man's body. He was alive. His heart pumped blood, his lungs took in air, thoughts came one after another. He could – in theory, anyway – laugh and love and continue meaningful relationships. So how would losing half his body alter his sense of self?

A Brazilian nursing student who spent time with thirteen patients before and after amputations described their experiences after losing a limb in surgery as 'living an incompleteness'. The amputees she followed wrestled with their new reality. They understood logically that their surgery was necessary but, emotionally, they did not accept the loss.

One thirty-one-year-old hemicorpectomy patient wrote heartbreakingly about his experience. Referred to only as Mr P, the patient had been thrown from a vehicle and paralysed at the age of eighteen. Over the next decade, he developed life-threatening pressure ulcers, prompting the drastic decision to remove the lower half of his body. After the surgery, he wrote personal essays in an attempt to come to terms with his new self:

> Staring at the night, I see the slate is not as blank as I thought. Before the night my old mental self stands face to face with my new physical self. The physical was no longer the death I feared but a future I embrace. I moved my hand downward from my chest across my belly button and my abdomen to my back, never lifting my hand. Stunned, I raised the sheets from my body and my head from the pillow. I cannot see the end of my body. My arm reaches out at an expanse of white – my mind is blank. There are no words to describe the loss. I drop the covers and my head, in tears. My physical self is no longer the problem . . .

Of the small number of people who have gone through hemicorpectomies since the surgery was devised in 1950, some have emerged with a renewed sense of purpose. There are reports of a patient studying for a Ph.D., of others still engaged in writing or photography. Sadly, I didn't see my patient again after he left the hospital. My part was done, and the general surgeons took over his care. I did, however, follow his progress. He struggled and, checking his medical notes, I found that he had had to be hospitalized months later for severe depression and suicidal ideation. My sense of regret grew. The psychological complications of a procedure are rarely considered by surgeons, but this patient's narrative was one I couldn't forget. Ever since, I never neglect to discuss with my patients the impact an operation may have on their sense of self.

The human brain has evolved not only to monitor the world around us but the world within. We are built to know whether we're hungry or cold, if we've stepped on a sharp piece of glass or our heart is racing. The brain is in a constant conversation with the rest of the body.

The brain even monitors what's going on within itself. None of this requires any effort: it's automatic. The act of sensing where our body is in space is called proprioception. The act of monitoring our psychological condition is called interoception, and incorporates not only the sensations themselves but how they are interpreted, regulated and acted upon. Interoception is at the heart of being human, of being aware of our feelings and emotions.

Problems with interoception can have profound consequences. People with xenomelia – literally, 'foreign limb' – believe that one or more of their limbs do not belong to them. This belief can be so powerful that people suffering from xenomelia want surgery in order to amputate the limb in question. For this reason, the condition was once called apotemnophilia ('love of amputation'). People with xenomelia can, however, live normal lives, hiding their belief that they live with a foreign limb.

The French philosopher Maurice Merleau-Ponty wrote that the body 'is our general medium for having a world'. When the body that walks or wears shoes is suddenly legless, he went on, there is a disconnect between the habit body and the present body. If the body is the medium for having a world, it's up to the brain to sort out that world. If our habitual sense of self and our present sense of self do not match, do we experience some sort of phantom self, a belief that the old self is still there?

Growing up, I never expected to be a surgeon. Unlike many of my peers in medical school and training, I did not have an all-consuming drive to become a physician from an early age. As a child in Los Angeles, I didn't imagine myself becoming any kind of careerist. I was no one's Most Likely to Succeed. Later, I dropped out of University of California, Berkeley, after a half-hearted effort, and took a job as a security guard at a Berkeley cafeteria. I wore a rent-a-cop uniform while watching my former classmates dine, their academic careers advancing. Mine appeared derailed.

When I decided to revive my college career to become a physician, advisers at college and university told me I was wasting my time. The consensus was that I had fallen too far to still have a shot at becoming part of the academic elite. After an unusual journey that took me through Compton Community College in South Central Los Angeles, it all took shape – university, medical school, graduate degree and a coveted slot in surgery.

I am a father, a surgeon, an Angelino. That's my identity. But what about my *self*? I've always considered myself unafraid to challenge conventional wisdom, to fight against the tide when necessary, as someone who puts the humanity of my patients above all else. That's what troubled me deeply about my role in this hemicorpectomy. I was a seasoned surgeon and I fell into the trap of going along with a group decision, with the course of action proposed by the 'multidisciplinary team', even though I could have argued for a less invasive approach. I'd allowed the group to intrude on my relationship with my patient, something I hold sacred. I'd acquiesced, even though my image of myself was that of a renegade. My present self was at odds with my habitual self, and it was tripping me up inside.

As we go through life, our sense of self, of who we are at the most fundamental level, rarely changes. This doesn't mean we can't learn and grow in profound ways. But what gives us this powerful sense of a unique self? For millennia, the answer to this question would have been the soul. In the last century, advances in science have led us to understand that the brain is the only possible answer. Neurophilosopher Patricia S. Churchland writes, 'It's our brain that creates our sense of self, our sense of being and individuality that persists through time.'

Our sense of self arises from an area of the brain called the insula, an island inside the brain's undulating, opalescent canopy of neurons, a canopy that ballooned so dramatically as we evolved that it had to fold itself like an accordion to fit into our skulls, hence its distinctive architecture. 'Insula' comes from the Latin word for 'island', and during the massive expansion of the ancient brain this island remained secret, tucked between the frontal and temporal lobes which give us our powers of reasoning and feeling. The insula is concealed in the brain and in turn conceals our inner selves.

For most of human history, the brain was a total enigma and explaining how it worked was the province of philosophers alone. It was only in the late nineteenth century that two great minds gave us the chance to see the human brain as an environment and ecosystem that evolves. The philosopher and psychologist William James described cognition as 'streams of thought' and the neurobiologist Santiago Ramón y Cajal, seeing neurons through his microscope, described them as 'mysterious butterflies of our soul'. Neither James nor Cajal characterized our brains as wires or wiring. Instead, they offered us the profound insight of understanding the brain as a living universe in which, throughout the course of our life, neurons are born from germinal niches of stem cells and their cellular fate is determined – literally – by our thoughts, emotions and intentions. These fundamental concepts are no less true today, and brain surgery, particularly when done when the patient is awake, is revealing a deeper insight into the ecology of our minds.

There are times when brain surgery directly places the insula, the guardian of the self, at risk. One such case was a patient who came to me with a rare manifestation of blood cancer. She had lymphoma, a white blood cell cancer which in her case formed in the central nervous system and remained defiant in the face of radiation therapy. The cancer had spread from the patient's blood to her brain. It was my job to surgically remove what cancer I could. The challenge was the location of the tumour: it was next to the insula.

Reaching the insula during surgery is not easy. Blood

vessels in the brain are not neatly packed cords; their layout is tortuous and serpentine and slightly different in each of us. These microvessels can tear if the caress of your instrument is coarse. You work top down, as if you are parting a tree's canopy to reach the thick branches deep inside. To get to the insula, you have to separate the frontal lobe from the temporal lobe. This space between the lobes is held together by the soft tug of overlapping blood vessels and a fine, opalescent membrane called the 'arachnoid', as it looks like a spider's web. The operating table was tilted at an angle so that the patient's head was lower than her feet. I parted the membranes and the two lobes fell apart, drawn by the gentle pull of gravity.

The tumour was unmissable. Its dull, coarse exterior lacked the glisten of healthy brain tissue. The hardest part of the dissection would take place underneath this clump of cancer, as the deepest section was nestled into the insula. It was a challenging procedure, and the most difficult point came at the very end, when fatigue can creep in. I created a plane between the tumour and the insula with a delicate scalpel on a long handle. The operation took several hours. Technically, it had gone well.

The next morning, I had seven patients to check on. I stopped by this patient's bed first. I always start with the sickest patients after surgery, just as I always start with the sickest patients during my operative day. She was on my mind because I had seen the island, been on the island, deep in her brain, that defined her *self*. And not only had I been to that island, I had removed poison from it.

When I arrived at her room, her feet were pointing towards a wall with a flatscreen TV on it. I approached from the left, and she greeted me immediately. She'd just had breakfast, and the sight of the food on her plate perplexed me. Imagine the plate as a clock. She had eaten the half that would come between six and twelve; the section between twelve and six remained untouched. When I walked over to the right side of her bed, she didn't acknowledge me; her head didn't even turn my way. What I was seeing was a rare case of right hemineglect: half of her body was invisible to her, as was half of her world. Brain scans done immediately after her surgery had shown that the tissue of the insula was perfectly intact. The patient was optimistic. By her own assessment, she was doing 'great'.

But something had happened with the tiny vessels that twist and turn in the bends that I had to navigate through during surgery. They are responsible for irrigating the ancient and essential island of self, the insular cortex. This was no split-brain stuff, not an example of the well-established phantom limb. Instead, the whole right half of the patient's universe was blocked from entering her mind. As it turned out, inflammation from the surgery near the insula had temporarily stunned the vital structure. This patient was shutting out half her body and the memory of her missing half. In that moment, I started to appreciate the extent to which our mind – not our brain – will go to keep a unified narrative of self.

The result was an incredibly deep defence mechanism, a coping mechanism beyond anything I had seen. It tore down my intellectual facade. Before that moment, I had thought I knew the brain and its magical creation – the human mind. Seeing how the mind can subdue its own flesh was something startling, but also revelatory. A few days later, the irritated neurons cooled off and my patient was completely herself and able to acknowledge the right-hand side of her body. However, she never fully came to grips with what had happened. To this day, she invents different stories to reconcile the inconsistencies in her remembered experience.

Sometimes, we come to understand our sense of purpose – our sense of *self* – in unexpected ways. There is a belief in my profession that death equals defeat. Physicians and surgeons are driven to go to extreme lengths – such as removing the lower half of a person's body – in order to save a patient's life. In training, I came to understand that my role was not always to save the patient's life. Sometimes, that simply wasn't possible. Sometimes, the most heroic thing I can do is bear some of the pain. I learned this early on in my career, through a severely injured child and her mother.

Before I saw them, I'd met the paediatric ICU physician in the hallway. Having put in over forty years, he was a veteran. He'd already experienced a lifetime of miracles and tragedies in the paediatric ICU. In a whisper, he'd told me the girl's condition. She had been hit by an SUV and was brain dead.

The girl was four. I was twenty-nine, a few years younger than her mother. I wanted to reassure the girl's mother that everything would be done as it should be for her daughter, but she was in a state of disbelief. Looking at the girl, you could see why. She wasn't shattered. She didn't have the patina of a paediatric cancer patient, with scars where ports had been built into them for drug infusions. She looked pretty normal, except for some scuffs, as though she'd fallen off her bike.

Her mother didn't believe that her daughter's lack of movement proved anything, nor did she believe the brain scans that showed no blood flow into the skull. Her daughter's heart was beating so hard its ripples could be felt with a finger on her wrist. The colour in her skin hadn't evaporated. She must have looked more or less the same when she woke up that morning. What proof did we have to let a warm, unbroken person go? I could see why a mother wouldn't take our word for it when her daughter's life was at stake.

Many children die after having been hit by a car, but usually their small bodies are shattered. So, in this

case, it was particularly hard for the mother to understand the extent of her daughter's injuries. She had
received 'that call' on her telephone answering machine.
This was before cellphones. Her nanny had left the
message: she was heading to the hospital because the
girl had been hit by a car. Imagine listening to that
recording.

I'd come down to the ICU but, this time, not to
help the child. No surgery could bring this girl back.
I'd been called in to play a role in a one-act tragedy
with three actors: a mother, a child, a surgeon. My
role was not to save the patient but something else
altogether, something where me taking a hit was part
of the equation. At the time, both the mother and I
were in the dark about our shared role in this drama.

The ICU old-timer had asked me to do something
that would make the girl's brain death incontestable
so that her mother could start to process the reality
and extent of her daughter's injuries. My part was to
make a small hole in her skull and take a brain pressure reading. To do that, I needed to place a thin,
flexible catheter into her cranial vault. This was to
show the mother that the pressure in her child's brain
was sky high, that no brain could survive under those
conditions. Looking back, he must have known that
the brain pressure numbers alone wouldn't convince
the girl's mother, but he'd asked me nonetheless. I
think he knew that the sound and sight of what I was
about to do would make the mother understand at

some awful, visceral level that her daughter was gone. I, too, was about to come to an understanding.

I'd been talking to this ICU physician for weeks about my desire to care for the sickest of the sick. I didn't enter medicine to write prescriptions, I'd told him. Maybe this was my test, my initiation rite. I'm only now coming to understand what happened, the weight he put on me.

I combed the girl's thin blonde hair as if I were a barber, giving her a right-side parting. Then I doused a little piece of gauze with alcohol and dabbed the crease. I loaded a syringe and squirted a little into the air. The syringe held nothing but saline. The girl wasn't going to need anaesthetic, but I wanted to fulfil my role in the ritual. Meet the expectation that everything was as it should be, as it had to be.

I had to make a tiny hole in the skull. The child didn't need any of this, but her mother did. She needed to know that things were done the way she anticipated after a lifetime of lies and the simplifications she'd seen on TV dramas. So, I moved forward, feeling in control of the scene, though I wasn't. No one asked what this was going to do to me.

The mother sat on the bed, holding her daughter's body on her lap. There were chalky streaks on her face from the salty residue of evaporated tears. She was in her office clothes. I was in my scrubs and put on sterile gloves. They are packed in paper and have to be put on in a particular way so you don't dirty the sterile exterior. From that moment on, everything was communicated through eye contact.

The mother had lived three decades, and her face had subtle lines, free of the furrows of a hard or long life. The look I saw on her face now was brand new. There were no creases to reveal that her face had ever made this expression before, and I had never seen anything like it. Contracting facial muscles had produced virgin valleys and shadows, creating a look of absolute pain. Pure grief. Pure disbelief. I could barely look her in the face. I could barely look away.

Back then, surgeons didn't wear face coverings or eye protection during bedside procedures. It's easy to conceal emotions behind the face masks and eye shields we wear now. No one sees the secret grimaces we make. But the only barrier between me and the situation that day were my scrubs and the surgical gloves. Both our faces – mine and the mother's – were exposed as we observed the unfolding tragedy and each other.

Her eyes were on her daughter's closed eyelids. On the dexterity with which I'd donned the gloves. My eyes glanced on her naked ring finger. I wondered where the girl's father was and if they had let him know what was about to happen. Her eyes as I punctured her daughter's tender scalp, so thin. No resistance. Her eyes watching not just my invasion but the confidence with which I was making it happen. 'No rookie' was the impression I needed her to walk away with. But I was. We can all spot a rookie from a fumble. That insight doesn't take medical training; it doesn't matter whether the surgeon has a tattoo or grey hair. I stabbed the scalp with a blade to make an opening the size of a fingernail in her flesh. The child didn't flinch, despite being on no sedation.

I prepared the drill, with its handle, egg-beater swivel and drill bit. It was a tool similar to one you might use to make a hole in a wall in order to pass a wire through, but in this case I was going to be passing a wire into her cranial vault – an electrical silicone wire designed to gauge the pressures in this vaunted space. The situation was grim. And now the girl's mother was watching my forearms, because the next steps weren't taken with fingertips. I turned the eggbeater handle with my right hand and held the drill's pistol grip steady with my left. The skull was familiarly hard, like rock, but when the drill tip penetrated and then entered the skull, just millimetres below, I could feel a pull on my left hand. I matched its gravitation by pulling backwards, opposing forces to keep from plunging in. This was a new feeling. Usually, it's soft, but the inside of a skull doesn't usually suck you in. It was as if the brain had a magnetic core. And then I revolved the egg-beater handle in reverse with my right hand and pulled out. The moment the drill was no longer plugging up the bony orifice, it happened.

The sound, like the hissing of air released from a punctured tyre, came first, and then the spray. Like a fine aerosolized mist, a carbonated fizz coated my face. The child's brain was morselized, evanescent, effervescent.

I was startled and disgusted all in a millisecond, but I knew the girl's mother was watching. I knew her child was gone, so I offered my condolences to the mother and child by not flinching, by not showing the sense of recoil I felt. By holding my position. My face and my body language were unwavering, my deepest emotions held at bay. I just blinked.

The last thing the mother needed was my disgust. I did redirect my gaze from the girl's head to the mother's face, without actually moving my head. My eyelids battled to not flutter but failed, as if they were automatic windshield wipers. Everything else, I caged, as the mother stood there in judgement. By not flinching, I could help the mother understand that every part of her child was sacred to me. I wanted to pause. I wanted to call for help. I wanted to be somewhere else, not here.

I persisted and dropped the catheter in. The reading was through the roof, as expected. It was irrelevant. No reasonable person could see their child's skull spew brain, like a whale expelling air through its blow hole, and not know the finality. The girl's mother did. I did. And now those extraterrestrial ridges and valleys on her face slowly flattened. She was depleted, exhausted, defeated. She let her daughter go a few hours later. And I was a different person.

I finished the procedure still with the mist on my face. It let her mother know that I respected her daughter's life and the gravity of what was happening. That's when I knew I was going to embrace this, this part of me that I wanted to have more of. That's the moment I knew I was meant for this work. It wasn't the hands, or the smarts, but the energy to tend to those more broken than I was. In that moment, I found out something unique about my *self*, so much truer than any label of 'physician' or 'surgeon'.

I went to the bathroom in the hallway of the hospital, still carrying the taste in my mouth and the mist in my eyes. I blinked, and breathed through my nose to avoid gulping the taste of her mind. But the smell wafted into my nose, olfaction going straight to my emotional brain. Thought can regulate all the senses but smell.

I splashed my face with water, wiped my face with coarse brown paper towels and went on with my day. That night, I hung out with my elder son, who at that time was a year old, saying nothing to his mother or anyone about what I had witnessed that day. Most of us keep our deepest, interior lives private. The residue of that experience hadn't faded and, frankly, it has never stopped reverberating.

Since then, I've wondered if the ICU physician knew in some strange way how the experience would affect me. Would it create in me a sense of self? I'd said I wanted to treat the sickest. Maybe this was his test to see if I was the rare trainee who meant it. Whether I was the one in a hundred who was ready, not only to put in the extra effort, skill and time but for the vicarious traumatization that comes from the inevitable bad outcomes. I've also wondered whether he called me down to the ICU because he intended to humble me in some way, rid me of some hubris. He set me up to absorb some of the mother's pain, but did he somehow know this experience would change the direction of my life, that this would be a moment that made me?

Each of us have a unique inner story, a sense of self born of our experience and beliefs, our memories and history, our hopes and desires. The ability to take episodes in our life and weave them into an ongoing narrative is called autobiographical memory, and it's the basis of how we see our *self*. Those mysterious butterflies that author our personal narrative tie our moments together. If self and autobiographical memory aren't on the same page, and memories fail to ground core beliefs, then people sprout delusions and even confabulations – as the patient with lymphoma dramatically showed after surgery around her insula.

Our autobiographical narrative can be challenged when we have to act in the face of adversity, when things happen that we never anticipated in our imagined future. The ability to weave these unpleasant events, these setbacks, these failures, into a narrative of purpose and some redemption is vital. We have a unique capacity to adapt our mental landscape to the challenges we face, to steer our stream of thoughts and determine our psychological fate. Coping is about protecting that continuity, that self-coherence of disparate life experiences. Coping is our toolkit for self-preservation.

Though I didn't talk about it at the time, that experience with the girl and her mother was now part of me. Until that moment, deep down, I wasn't sure I wanted to be a physician. I'd dropped out of college then clawed my way back to college and into medical school because I felt I should. My experience with this tragically injured girl and her mother revealed something new about me – to me. I surprised my *self.* Only in that crucible did something more profound surface about me. Strangely, it was a gift, a secret I shared only with myself: I discovered I was capable of self-control. I felt the first inklings of a self-worth that transcended my professional identity, something inside me I wanted to protect, cultivate and rely upon when I was faced with life's difficulties.

4.

Failure

The evening Karina's legs didn't come alive, I could see her future clearly. When I got that call from the nurses a few hours after surgery had been completed, I was hoping the problem was only that the narcotics from the anaesthesia hadn't cleared. Karina's legs weren't moving, but patients often don't respond evenly immediately after surgery. Sometimes, arms and legs reanimate differently, as though the patient is drunk. So I asked the questions: Had she woken up from the anaesthesia? The nurse said she was wide awake. Do her arms move? I was dreading the response I could feel was coming.

I called the operating theatre for an emergency take-back. A take-back is a return to the operating room for the same patient in under twenty-four hours. Nothing blares 'surgeon error' more than a take-back. I unravelled the stitches I'd made just a few hours ago to reopen the cut. Everyone, including the girl's parents, could sense the disaster. I knew what had happened because, during the surgery, I'd had to choose one of two routes I could have taken to end the surgery. It was a thought that had floated in my mind, a possibility of failure. The decision I made was to do less in the closing steps of surgery. Doing less work would make the surgery quicker, reducing the chances of complications such as infection, but leaving a possibility that the girl's spine might be less sturdy. Instinct had been telling me to take the second, longer route. Yet I didn't. I went for the quicker surgery. The decision I made was justifiable on paper, but I had ignored my gut and made the wrong choice. An unfixable mistake – a burden surgeons inevitably have to bear.

Karina was eleven years old, old enough for me to be able to explain why we were meeting to her as well as to her parents. I first met the three of them in a children's hospital, decorated as they always are like a macabre Disneyland, with bright colours and cartoon figures among the children. Karina was in possession of a calm and poise often not found even in adults. She was an old soul. Her parents had a positive energy, a devout couple who had finally found parenthood and a deeply fulfilling life by adopting Karina. They told me they could tell in an instant by the way the three of them looked at each other that they were her parents and she was their child. Biology was superfluous. The connection was profound, spiritual and regenerative.

Karina stood out to me from the outset because she had something called diastematomyelia. As she grew, her spinal cord was being glacially split down the middle, slowly bisected by a piece of errant bone that protruded backwards from the vertebrae and into the bony tunnel that houses the brain's exquisitely sensitive tail, the spinal cord. The bony keel had split the spinal cord, but the gradual growth of childhood meant that this had so far occurred only in one spot in the middle of her back, like a giant wave around a lighthouse.

The unanticipated dimple and buckled skin on the middle of her spine had alerted the paediatricians to look deeper. An MRI had shown a stalactite of bone right on the midline. Just as we have a left brain and a right brain, there is a left- and right-sidedness to our spinal cord. This is why this girl was, for now, still perfect. Only the midline was split, in a tiny spot. She would most likely be fine, as long as the keel didn't grow – or she didn't grow.

Puberty was around the corner, though, and Karina would certainly grow, and grow fast. A burst of height could tear the spinal cord vertically stretching against the immoveable bony keel: a vertical guillotine. As she grew taller, the keel would rip the cord beneath it, which would paralyse Karina's legs. It wouldn't be a sideways curvature of the spine like scoliosis, which sometimes happens in adolescent girls and is usually managed with a brace or, on occasion, surgery. This would be something more nefarious. The keel would essentially be a blade that cut her spinal cord down the middle. That's why she was referred to me. She and her parents met me to discuss whether they should take a wait-and-see approach or get in there and shave the shark tooth down so the spinal cord could stretch unimpeded. Both options carried risks, but her parents were optimistic.

Cases like Karina's are in many ways more difficult than trauma. In trauma, people come in injured and desperately need immediate treatment. Patients like Karina walk in perfect and the surgeon has to weigh up the risks of doing nothing against the risks of performing surgery. It's a judgement call based on a fraught calculus: which option is more likely to end badly.

Karina was my first case of the day. What happened to her wasn't a failure to execute a surgical manoeuvre. This wasn't about my hands or my technique. My failure was the product of both a loss of vigilance and not allowing my instincts to have their say.

When the skin is cut and the muscles are parted left and right, the spine looks like a lobster tail. The segmented and shingled bony rings allow for protection and movement. The bony protuberances you can feel running down your back are not the spine but the strange vestigial features of dinosaurs, a stegosaurus, maybe. They are like a mohawk on the spinal column, a decorative crest that can be clipped without issue. Four inches deep into the skin is a bony tunnel, the spinal canal. There, you'll find the spinal cord, the light-speed communication cables between the brain and the body. Sever or damage these gossamer fibres and the consequences can be both profound and – almost always – irreversible.

The spinal cord is a long, delicate structure and the material in it is the same as in the brainstem. It is the tail of the reptilian brain and, like the brain, it is housed in bone and ensconced in the same sheath, the dural sheath. The brain and spinal cord both float in the same cerebrospinal fluid. Pathways in the spinal cord look like the folds of a delicate curtain and when you surgically expose the spine's segmented lobster tail, vertical windows can be drilled or chiselled into it. The pieces of bone are then lifted and set aside on the back table.

In Karina's case, I'd carved out the roof of the spinal column with a fine drill in case I decided to replace the bones during the closure. With a sharp knife, I made a vertical incision on the dura covering her spinal cord. The two halves of the dural sheath were held apart with delicate stitches to the muscles that had been separated. The spinal cord is a beauty. You can see serpentine vessels on the back of the bright white, glistening cord. In fact, it's whiter than the brain, which has neuronal cell bodies that look bluish grey in the cortical canopy. The spinal cord is mostly tentacles, long extensions from the brain's neurons that carry signals. These were all tightly tucked electrical highways, and the surface showed the fine ridges.

Karina had been lying face down on the operating table when I removed the piece of spinal column. From this perspective, I thought of it as the roof of her spine. To get her out of the operating room, though, she'd need to be flipped on to her back, and the weight of her body would rest on the spot that had been removed and replaced. This spot would therefore have to bear her weight. The roof of the spinal column would then become the base, the foundation. The thought crossed my mind that Karina's spine would need more support. Should I buttress and fortify the closure to ensure there were no grave complications, or should I let it be so that she wouldn't have to deal with the additional risks that come with extra work? Should I do more or less? The question often comes up in the surgeries I do. More means more risk, usually, but less means the patient is exposed to a different palette of injuries. There are risks in doing something, and risks in not doing something. I'd thought about this during Karina's surgery and I'd decided on less. But when I got that call from the nurses, I knew I had made the wrong call. It was an error in judgement that had left her vulnerable.

When Karina was flipped from her stomach to her back her spinal column settled into itself: the spinal canal collapsed where I had opened the window for surgery. The result was an imploding tunnel. What was inside that tunnel – her spinal cord – was crushed. When I learned that her legs didn't move after surgery, I knew what had happened. I understood the physiology of the injury, the anatomy of preventable devastation. During the take-back, I lifted off the settled, crushing bone, but the damage to the spinal cord was already done. There was no fixing this mistake. Opening her up a second time confirmed what I already knew, and my dread solidified into something real and permanent, a failure that would change Karina, her parents and me.

The morning after the surgery, the social workers and nurses were doing their best to keep Karina feeling positive, despite the obvious weight of the calamity. Nothing had changed from the night before, when I received the call from the nurses. Karina reported that her legs were numb, but numbness is in fact a sensation. It's the feeling of loss.

Karina sat with a blanket from home covering her lifeless legs. A nurse on a break had brought a beach ball into the room. She would throw it to Karina, and Karina would throw it back. The room was quiet – no noisy machines, none of the frenzy of the operating room or the ICU, just one pole with a few drips. She was receiving intravenous steroids for the spinal cord injury, as she would had she fallen off a horse or crashed a motorcycle. The room had an uncommon configuration, with the window behind her head rather than to the side, and Karina's face was in silhouette. I was glad about that, because I was dreading the look in her eyes.

Karina was so young she couldn't imagine much past the moments in front of her. Her parents were people with deep faith who trusted in the future. I could see the future – hers and theirs – but not mine. Karina's legs would never move and would, over time, wither and contort. Her bladder would stop working and fill with infections. A hole would have to be made above her vagina as a port to drain her bladder. A bag on her abdominal wall would collect her faeces. Her genitals would shrivel and be insensate, despite puberty. Would she develop life-threatening pressure ulcers? Her parents couldn't imagine this future. What parent could?

Karina's demeanour didn't change. She didn't break from the equanimity she had before surgery. I was spared from seeing her eyes as the light from the window was shining on mine. I was feeling so much. Shame. Self-loathing. Failure. I needed to rein in those emotions to provide some reassurance, a reassurance based on an extremely low chance of her ever walking. Since, on the rare occasion, a patient or two have recovered enough to walk with braces, I took that 1 per cent statistic as licence to offer some hope to the family. I told them what was easiest for all of us in that room to hear.

Karina's parents were more than kind. They understood the grave consequences and complications that come with choices made in surgery. Never once did the parents look at me with the hate, the disgust, the wrath, I had earned. They remained steadfast in their faith that this was part of a higher purpose. How they came to find her. How she filled their spirit. They were forgiving, accepting, tolerant, deeper, stronger than me. All the things I was not. All the things I couldn't be. The day they left the hospital I didn't even go to see them. I could have made time, but I was glad there was surgery scheduled so I could save face. The shame was unconcealable.

I was a coward. I remember her parents telling me how Karina filled them with life, an emotional depth and complexity that hadn't existed before. What I had done during surgery would test that depth with the challenge of a life in a wheelchair, a life in the tragic wake of my individual failure. I'd made a judgement call despite the dissenting voice, my instinct, telling me to do something else.

I felt a shame that undermined my sense of self and the narrative I had created that I was talented at this craft I had chosen as my career. I was guilty of making the wrong mistake, the unfixable complication in the list of surgical complications. It's said that shame grows with secrecy. This was no secret. It took place under the unforgiving fluorescent lights of the operating room, and the whole hospital knew. My shame cast an ugly shadow on the identity I had worked hard to build, both internally and externally. I felt like a fraud. That experience cut deep. A beating would have been more healing, would have been more welcome than this.

What does it take to get past an irreversible mental lapse? When Karina's case was presented at M&M, the weekly Morbidity and Mortality meeting where all the surgeons assemble, it was a strange confessional, but I didn't feel that my sins had been purged or cleansed. I stood in front of my peers and detailed my mistakes and the thinking that had led to them. My peers let me off easy for my 'error of judgement', following the established practice of protecting one of their own. I should have been held closer to the flame, scorched a bit. I should have been scarred professionally, demoted, relegated to something probationary, but the system protected itself by calling what happened to Karina a 'complication' rather than an error.

I knew right away the physical challenges Karina would be facing in the months and years ahead, but I started to wonder about the mental hurdles. How would her sense of self be altered by paralysis? Would she grieve with her parents over the loss of her legs? The brain is not floating alone and independent in a vat of cerebrospinal fluid. It is connected to the body and in constant communication with it. Just like the man who underwent a hemicorpectomy, Karina's body had changed profoundly.

I felt like I had got away with something, and it ate at me. It festered inside me, picked at and frayed the loose threads of the narrative of self I'd spent years weaving. The experience became a barrier, keeping me from feeling satisfied or happy. I knew I shouldn't have had second thoughts about my second thoughts. I should have trusted those instincts.

After Karina, I felt surrounded by gloom, with the perpetually sunny skies of Los Angeles a constant taunt. My mental state was the opposite of that of the French writer Albert Camus, who said, 'In the depths of winter, I finally learned that within me lay an invincible summer.' In the invincible LA summer, I was enduring my own private winter. At our darkest moments, the thing we believe least is that things will change – could change. Like some of my patients, I learned to lie with my eyes, feign with my face, because I wanted to conceal my interior life. I didn't want to have to explain the inexplicable.

For me, this period of despair eventually brought a profound change, a broadening of my empathy and a widening of my perceptions of others who were also privately suffering. Failure served as an asset in my understanding of the world and other people's vulnerabilities. Some physicians develop empathy fatigue. I was experiencing a new reservoir of empathy. The struggle created a humility in me. I saw the world differently. I saw others' emotions more clearly. In my suffering, there was a chance for me to belong, a chance for patients who were also suffering to see in me that I, too, bore a burden. Now, we could talk openly.

My cancer patients do not have the luxury of the double life I was living, a public self and a private torment. Their diagnosis is known to those around them. Some of them tell me they hate it when people ask how they are doing and find the 'you can do it' pep talks only add to their anguish. Most cancer patients experience emotional distress. Knowing the existential challenge of a cancer diagnosis, some hospitals now offer therapy through behavioural oncology programmes, helping patients with feelings of panic, sadness, anger, guilt and hopelessness.

But I had hang-ups about getting help, as I was aware it wasn't something surgical comrades would see as brave. Quite the opposite: anyone who showed any kind of vulnerability was considered weak. I had my own biases, too. Even though psychiatrists had been to medical school and could prescribe meds, they were on the bottom of our respect totem pole. Still, psychiatrists were trained physicians. A psychiatrist in training suggested a book to me after my poorly concealed, easily deciphered reach for guidance. He suggested *An Unquiet Mind: A Memoir of Moods and Madness*, by Kay Redfield Jamison, a professor of psychiatry. In it, she writes, 'My body is uninhabitable. It is raging and weeping and full of destruction and wild energy gone amok.' I could relate.

With Karina, here's what I should have done. I should have taken the time to place some screws to fortify her spine where I'd opened the window into the spinal canal rather than returning the bones I'd removed. I had put the lid back on the jar, but the lid was barely wide enough to bridge the jar's opening. The thought had crossed my mind that the free-floating bone wouldn't perch on her spine and could settle into the canal where the delicate cord lay. I could have added in tiny screws to make sure the lid was actually re-attached to the jar, to the tunnel.

I had options how to close this box, and I chose the wrong one. I remember vividly running through the reasoning, the pros and cons, of what to do, and I still live with that error in judgement. This was a complication that didn't have to happen. I didn't say to myself: Make the move that ensures she doesn't have the worst possible complication of this surgery. This is what matters most and what should drive decisions most. I got caught up in my own thoughts. I went academic. Never again. I won't make that mistake again.

We all fail. We all have moments in our lives we wish could be unlived or relived. This is the nature of being human. I took to the admonition Samuel Beckett included in his novella *Worstward Ho*: 'Ever tried. Ever failed. No matter. Try again. Fail again. Fail better.' I'd love to redo Karina's surgery from the beginning, but I can't. It doesn't work that way. I did want to set what had happened to her right in some way, and so I've tried to replace my failure with performance and skill: hurting people less than the other masters of my profession. The risk can never get to zero, but I want to be the one closest to that number. Of all the events of my life, this one experience shook me the most. There are things we can do to reduce the chance of our traumatic memories becoming consolidated, from following us and injecting themselves into our daily lives. I didn't do any of them at the time. Time heals nothing if we don't permit it to.

Advances in knowledge, in medicine and in life come through failure, with success arriving bruised but victorious on the back of ignorance, rejection, loss, frustration, pain and death. To play it safe, to take no chances, to enter the fray trying not to lose and living not to fail is a recipe for stagnation and not much of a life at all. To step forward, we have to be willing to misstep.

Failure does not have to sow self-doubt, unflattering self-evaluation and fear. Even though failure is universal, it is largely hidden from view. Psychology professor Johannes Haushofer upended this convention when he published a 'CV of Failures', listing the programmes he didn't get into and the academic positions and fellowships he didn't get. At the top of his CV, beneath his name, Haushofer wrote, 'Most of what I try fails, but these failures are often invisible, while the successes are visible. I have noticed that this sometimes gives others the impression that most things work out for me.'

There are many ways to fail. Some are beneficial. The basketball player Michael Jordan was acutely aware of every failure, and that gave him the ammunition to learn and grow. Jordan said, 'I've missed more than 9,000 shots in my career. I've lost almost 300 games. Twenty-six times, I've been trusted to take the game-winning shot and missed. I've failed over and over and over again in my life. And that is why I succeed.'

The history of medicine, too, is largely one of failure, of trial and error, of learning from mistakes. The advances arrive as the result of its failings, not in spite of them. For surgeons, the goal is to improve our skills and our knowledge as we work to make failure as infrequent as possible. We want to make failure an endangered species, a rare sighting, and when we do fail, we want our shortcomings to be as trivial as possible. If we fall short in the operating theatre, we want it to be a hard landing rather than a crash.

Too often, death itself is considered a failure. We are trained to take heroic action to save even the oldest, sickest patient. That puts surgeons, including me, in a strange position. Of the last thousand cancer patients who put their trust in me, all died within a few years of meeting me. I operate on incurable cancer – stage 4. There is no stage 5. But I'm not a failure, despite the statistics.

As a cancer surgeon who cares for patients in whom breast cancer has spread to the brain or spine, most of my patients are women. Stage 4 breast cancer means the cancer has spread from its origin to different organs. Many of these patients have survived their first bout with breast cancer, only to have it come back, spread and evolve a more aggressive biology. Jane was one such patient.

Looking at the MRI of Jane's brain, I saw a large white circle on the image, a massive tumour that had caught Jane by surprise. She thought she had beaten cancer. Scans of her breast and body had been negative, and she was back working as a nurse and living a full life when she started having difficulty concentrating. Her typing slowed. In her own words, she thought she was 'cracking up'. She went to see a psychiatrist, thinking she had lost her mind, but after the MRI she came to me.

In the United States, there are more than 23,000 cancer cases every year where the cancer has originated in the brain or the spinal cord. Glioblastoma is one such cancer. Twenty times more common are cancers such as Jane's that spread to the brain from the breast, lungs or another part of the body. Jane's cancer cells had escaped her breast years ago and had now colonized her brain. I removed her brain tumour, and subsequent brain scans showed that it was gone. However, cancer was not yet done with Jane.

Jane lived for four years after I removed a giant ball of malignant breast cancer tissue from her brain. The tumour had been in one of her occipital lobes, so she lost only opposite peripheral vision, meaning she could still drive, she just couldn't trust her left wing mirror when she did. During those four years, Jane saw her children marry, and the birth of a grandchild. However, on one of her visits to the hospital, I looked at Jane's smile and it worried me. It didn't pull up evenly. The corners of her mouth were like marionette strings, but with one string failing to pull. It looked like she was smirking. This was harmless enough. What worried me was what I suspected lay behind the lopsided smile. I feared that one of the cranial nerves from her brain towards her face was coated with cancer cells, making the signals slow and causing them to drop out – like trying to make a cellphone call with spotty reception. If that was the case, there would be cancer cells in the fluid in which the brain floats. That fluid would have to be sampled for testing.

Later that week, Jane lay in a foetal position on a hospital bed as I set to work creating an opening in the shingling bones of her spine. I slid a needle into her lower back, between the bones and the longitudinal ligament that connects them, then through the dural sheath, and the nerves slithered away, as fish do when you step into a stream. The spinal cord stops in the lowest part of the back and splits into individual nerves that look like a horse's tail, allowing safe withdrawal of cerebrospinal fluid with a spinal tap. This is the same fluid that circulates in the brain. I was going to withdraw a small amount of fluid and send it off to the lab to discover if a pathologist could see any cancer cells under the microscope. Even finding one cancer cell would mean that Jane had the diagnosis of carcinomatous meningitis. If the pathologist found this cell, it would mean Jane's tumour had spread to the meninges, thin layers of tissue that line and protect the brain and spinal cord. This fluid is clear – or it's supposed to be. Jane's wasn't. Far from it. She had so many cancer cells her spinal fluid was cloudy, like those snow globes you buy in a gift shop. This was the worst-case scenario. This wasn't snowfall in London but radioactive ash falling over Chernobyl.

Jane had beaten the odds for four years despite the cancer having spread to her brain, so she was grateful. She had been living on borrowed time. She felt calm and joyful to have outlived the expectations she'd built many years before she met me, with her primary medical oncologists. In fact, when she came to see me, her first reaction was surprise. Why would a woman with breast cancer ever end up in a brain surgeon's clinic?

So throughout those years, she and I talked about a fate already established, a destination already locked in. She was stage 4. We had time to get to know each other, to discuss along the way what was inevitable, but the story of the end remained unforeseeable. Would her cancer spread to her liver, to other areas? Would there be other complications? There are lots of ways to go. We never talked about carcinomatous meningitis, but we did talk about a gracious ending that she could design herself.

When I saw that weird asymmetric smile, I let Jane know what I was thinking. When the fluid was cloudy, I spoke to her after she turned over from the foetal position. This wasn't information she wanted me to hold back and parse out in a separate clinic visit. She wanted to know, had a right to know. She could tell from my face. I didn't really need to say anything. That's what patients read – not your words, but your energy. She took a deep breath and smiled, crookedly.

A few minutes later, having composed herself, she said, 'In your trusted hands, we shall try to make it to Christmas.' When Jane spoke of my hands, she was speaking metaphorically. She knew surgery was not an option. It was summertime, and she realized that her remaining life would be measured in months, but we were still hopeful we could push that statistic back, as we did when she had brain cancer and people said she had only a year.

In my dreams for months afterwards I was obsessed with the biological narrative of how breast cancer can spread into the brain's bony aquarium. This is the worst place for cancer to spread. Some people with a stage 4 diagnosis live for decades. Many live for years. When any cancer spreads to the cerebrospinal fluid, patients have only months. No matter where your cancer originates, when it enters the fluid around your brain and spinal cord you have carcinomatous meningitis, a diagnosis that makes even cancer specialists want to throw in the towel. You can feel the hush and deflation in veteran cancer physicians when they hear this diagnosis.

In the past, we didn't offer patients like Jane, whose cancer had spread to the brain, any real treatment. Traditionally, such cases were considered hopeless. Even today, many medical physicians would call Jane's original brain surgery aggressive, as many physicians elect not to operate on cancer that has spread to the brain. I didn't think it was aggressive, and neither did she. Then, when she asked me what to do about this deepest malignant invasion, the cancer in her cerebrospinal fluid, I said something that many medical physicians would have thought inappropriately passive. I said, 'Maybe nothing at all,' because Jane had always urged me to let her know 'when to walk away'. I used to tell her, 'We'll get there together,' and she would shake her head and reiterate, 'When I need to walk away, I want you to make the call.'

The conversation about letting go happened when her medical oncologists, her breast cancer specialists, admitted Jane to evaluate her for the medical issues. They were offering her palliative chemotherapy, which might make you feel better but cannot make you live longer. She knew that more chemotherapy to feel better made little sense for her as a person. For her plans, for herself. While in the hospital, she asked me, 'Is it time?' I nodded my head twice and she gave a single nod back and took a deep breath. In the slow exhalation, there was resolution. Cancer's march is indefatigable.

In the conversation with Jane there was one more subject I wanted to raise. I wanted to know whether she was willing to undergo one final operation, only hours after her death. This was not an easy conversation, but it was one I was having with other stage 4 cancer patients. Their cancer had sown the seeds of its own demise, running out of space to grow. In each case, the cancer would kill its host – my patients. But even after their death, the cancer itself would live for another six hours, giving us a small window to dissect the tumours.

Once these samples have been collected, we can grow these cell cultures indefinitely in the lab. Because cases like Jane's were, traditionally, considered beyond hope, little research has been done on metastatic breast cancer and not enough tissue had been collected over the years. I wanted to change that. Many patients with stage 4 cancer who feel there has been no purpose in the cancer literally consuming them do not flinch at the thought of a rapid autopsy after their deaths. Their bodies had failed them, but their minds hadn't. Jane was all in.

Hours after death, if the patients have agreed to let us collect tissue samples, all of their organs are removed and samples taken. We are interested in the mutations the breast cancer cells have undergone that allow them to colonize varied landscapes inside their world, the body. When we've removed the organs, we stitch up the scalp, chest, belly and pelvis so there is still the option of an open casket at the funeral. It may seem macabre, but Jane wanted to help. For her, it was an opportunity. A legacy.

Though we failed to save Jane, she will help save others from metastatic cancer. Jane wanted her tissue to be used to facilitate the invention of new medicine. In my laboratory, we are studying Jane's cells and those taken from other patients to decipher how cancer cells move from one part of the body to another. How do rogue breast cancer cells escape the organ of their origin and travel to other organs? How do the cancer cells then invade those organs, take root there? Can we find cancer's biological Achilles heel? Once you understand something, you can knock it down.

The failure with Jane became a different kind of engine than Karina. Less intense and more construct-ive, putting failure to good use. From failure, you can learn. From defeat, you can still plot a way forward. In the aftermath of Karina's surgery, I needed to learn and find my way forward. That took time and would lead me to challenge myself as a surgeon in ways, at least initially, that were not healthy.

One thing I wouldn't change is how I guided Karina and her parents after surgery, saying that there might be a small chance she could walk again. After over a

decade of carrying out cancer surgery, I would probably say the same thing to her now. Back then, I said
it because I was afraid. I did it for myself. Now, I think
a glimmer of hope is needed when you drop such a
bombshell. As the weeks go by in the hospital, and as
the patients are bracing themselves and adjusting to
the situation minute by minute, day by day, they
begin to see for themselves the unlikelihood that
things will improve. A rare patient will recover, or at
least preserve bowel and bladder function, and a
degree of hope seems to help patients push through
the arduous weeks ahead. With Karina, I was trying
to protect myself from the horrible reality of what
had happened, but I felt that giving her and her parents some hope was also the right thing to do for
them. I reached out, but I never heard from Karina or
her family again. I was left to imagine their reality
and deal with my failure alone.

When the boot heel of failure pushes you down,
how you get back up is the important thing. Life's
invariable failures, whether personal or professional,
can be a source of motivation, drive and growth.
Karina's case was for me – it pushed me to be better,
to keep learning and striving for improvement.

5.

Belief

The steep ascent from sea level had me gently clutching the right armrest. The window seat gave a view of stunning peaks, a distraction from the dangerous drop that needed to be made. Climbing out of Lima, Peru, was easy, but the pilots would have to land the passenger jet on an airstrip that seemed more suited to helicopters. The runway at El Alto airport near La Paz, Bolivia, looks like a tabletop sitting inside an extinguished volcano. The hot and high conditions there require a high-speed approach. Everyone else on board was local and composed, despite the jarring descent.

When we touched down, my left temple popped as though it had been hit with a ball-peen hammer. The pain at the upper outer edge of my eye socket caught me by surprise. I touched my temple with the pad of my finger, half expecting blood from bumping my head against the side of the cabin. It was dry. I realized the pain wasn't from outside my head, it was from inside, a drilling migraine from having climbed to more than 11,500 feet in, essentially, an instant after being at sea level on the South American west coast.

I knew why my head ached: it was because of my lungs. My chest was heaving because the air was so thin and my cerebral arteries were throbbing as a result.

In 2002, I went to La Paz to meet Jorge, the head of their only children's hospital. I remember that trip not just because of the migraine and the steep descent but because of the deep impact what I experienced there had on me. I didn't know it when I arrived, but I'd be involved in a surgery that would reshape my understanding of belief. Jorge and I had connected on email when I reached out to collaborate and try to equip their hospital with modern surgical tools. At the airport, he looked past me, expecting someone older. Even in the sparsely populated space, he'd missed me. I was young. I had a hoodie on, so no surprise he had trouble picking out 'Dr' Jandial among the arriving passengers. He was wearing a jacket with a Hospital del Niño badge on it. I approached him, and we started talking shop. We still laugh with our families when he tells that story.

The airport sits on the *altiplano*, the high plain above La Paz. The precipices were so steep into this ancient city, built on the inner jagged ridges of a cauldron trellised by cable cars. In a reversal of the way most cities are laid out, the poor are sequestered to the highest ground, giving them the best views but an onerous climb to get home if they can't afford the cable car.

Jorge and I went for a walk on the serpentine roads.

As we walked, I spotted two dead rats, or so I thought. Something wasn't quite right, though. As I got closer, I realized they weren't rats at all but the furry bodies of two bats with their heads missing. I asked Jorge what animal had done this. His face reflected my naivety back at me. He pointed to the clean cut on the neck, made by a blade. Not animals, he said, but humans.

He said it was *medicina amazonia*. Bat's blood and belief. Bolivians buy live bats in the marketplaces in order to drink fresh bat blood; they believe it has healing properties, especially an ability to manage seizures. That's the belief. It's not legal, nor does any data back it up, but sprinkle in the sporadic nature of seizures and you can come away with the impression that any pause in a seizure is connected to drinking bat's blood, not the result of chance. Cessation after intervention implies causality – if it is evaluated on the slippery slopes of belief. However, Jorge didn't disparage believers in *medicina amazonia*. Changing their understanding would take time, he said. We would have to show them that medicine – even the limited medicine available in La Paz – can help.

Both ancient and modern medicine are built on a foundation of hope. Whether people believe in the efficacy of bat's blood or brain surgery, hope gives patients a feeling that they have some influence on the present and a reason to plan for the future. In the face of isolation, pain or uncertainty, hope is an ally. Jorge introduced me to the patient I was there to see,

Chico, whose literal and figurative world had become very unstable. He needed hope.

Chico – the name is a term of endearment that means 'young man' – was an experienced labourer and his family's main breadwinner, but he was also only fifteen years old – a boy, in some respects. Kindly but firmly, Jorge spoke to him: 'We must face this fate unflinchingly.' He spoke to Chico as though he were asking an older man for surgical consent. At his age, Chico should still have something juvenile about him, but his hands showed that he had been working for years. And they revealed something else: a clue about his illness.

Jorge asked Chico to tell him what number he was drawing on the palm of his hand – the sharp lines of the number 7 or the curves of an 8, the verticality of 1 versus the pattern of a 3 – but when the teenager looked away, he had no idea. Finger agnosia. Patients with finger agnosia can read Braille with their finger-tips, they can decipher a number you make in the air, but not when someone else's finger traces the number on their palm. His hand was a window to his mind, guiding us to suspect his left hemisphere was the origin of his seizures. Chico was also deeply religious, and this hyper-religiosity was another clue that his seizures originated in the temporal lobe.

Chico's EEG showed temporal lobe epilepsy and a scan showed hamartoma, a non-cancerous tumour, a strange malformed tuft of his brain's cortex. The cortical canopy is thin but complex, with six pre-scribed microscopic layers, a vertical architecture like vines ascending to different heights. The vines are neurons, and the layers they reach are determined by whether they are receiving signals from elsewhere in the cortex, from the opposite hemisphere, or from the brainstem and spinal cord. Chico's hamartoma had thrown these layers into disarray, as though he had tilled this part of the brain's garden. As a result, neurons were firing off the wrong layers. This lack of cohesion was an electrical storm disturbing the normal signalling. When this happened, Chico suffered a partial seizure – partial because it involved only part of his brain.

Partial seizures were a part of Chico and part of how he was known locally. These episodes made Chico appear to stare blankly, and some in the community said Chico's sight was turned inwards to God. Chico faced no stigma because of his epilepsy. He began to cherish it. Welcome it, even. What he gleaned from those apparently blank stares, that dimension inside his mind, made him connect with nature in the Amazon, with God and his local church. And Chico had become a bit of a celebrity because of this.

Epilepsy has long been linked to religious fervour, ecstatic mystical experiences and visions of the divine. Some believe the profound religious experiences of Joan of Arc had their origin in epilepsy or seizures. She described being inspired by voices and visions, accompanied by 'a great light'. Joan of Arc said that she had first experienced a voice from God when she was thirteen, in her father's garden, and that, initially, she was frightened. Scholars now believe she may have had temporal lobe epilepsy.

A temporal lobe seizure may also have prompted the religious conversion of St Paul. On the road to Damascus, 'suddenly a light from heaven flashed round him; he dropped to the ground'. When he arose, he was blind for three days. In a letter to the Church of Corinth, Paul wrote that he experienced 'visions and revelations' and felt 'caught up to paradise and heard sacred secrets no human lips can repeat'. At the time, he said, he was unsure if he was 'in the body or out of the body'. Known for his prolific writing, Paul may have experienced another side effect of temporal lobe epilepsy: hypergraphia, an intense desire to write or draw.

A small number of patients with temporal lobe epilepsy report having had religious experiences. Patients report being in God's presence, hearing God's voice and experiencing salvation. The wellspring of Chico's religious visions prompted a medical diagnosis, suggesting abnormal biology, but for him it had been something to cherish. Belief resides in the chemical, molecular and electrophysiological spaces of the brain and integrates seamlessly with other currents within us: reward and arousal.

Over and over, I've seen faith act as a comforting

companion to my patients on their cancer journey. On the morning of their cancer surgeries, nearly all of my patients are embraced and comforted by faith. It also helps them shape a narrative of their experience, no matter how grim. And faith gives hope, which helps patients persevere. Faith and hope are inseparable – and invaluable in the face of cancer.

Before Chico, the depth and power of a patient's faith was something I didn't understand. I was naive, sceptical. Chico, on the other hand, didn't question his faith. He simply accepted his transcendent moments as a welcome part of his life. His deep connection to a profound spiritual world was coming to an end, however, as the result of worsening seizures and the surgery he would need.

Work was not a choice for Chico. To me, he was still a boy as he was only fifteen, but he was a man in this terrain, working the land to provide for his family. Then he fell. And fell again. The partial seizures turned to general seizures, ricocheting across cerebral landscapes, leading to sudden loss of consciousness. And that made him concerned, not for himself, but for his ability to keep working, for his family, his village. Now it had gone too far and he came to Hospital del Niño.

When I heard Jorge and Chico talking, I got the sense Chico had self-tapered, deliberately taking himself off his medication. 'Self-tapering' is a way for some patients to communicate that they like their mind as it is – unreined, un-numbed, unsated by medication that might quell not only aberrant electricity but also the sparks that make life deep and thrilling. Chico didn't want to take the pills but, now, even reintroducing them was not keeping him from falling. His mind was feral again, and when he passed out he didn't wake with the clarity and connection he cherished. This was what he missed most. That's why he was worried about the surgery. Not about surviving the opening of his skull, but whether his connection with the ethereal would endure.

Some patients will self-taper their psychiatric medications because they like the wild swings, the access to bigger neurotransmitter waves to surf. Bipolars self-taper; sober people self-taper off sobriety. Like them, Chico didn't want to take medication. It wasn't that it was costly or a burden on his family. He liked the way those partial seizures and in-between moments made him feel, and not just feel, but connect to something outside his inner feelings and interior life.

Like Chico, Fyodor Dostoyevsky had epilepsy but didn't like the anti-seizure medicine of his day, potassium bromide. The writer may also have self-tapered to embrace his ecstatic state just before a seizure, an aura, a moment when he experienced 'a happiness unthinkable in the normal state and unimaginable for anyone who hasn't experienced it . . . I am then in perfect harmony with myself and the entire universe.'

Such a transcendent feeling must have given

Dostoyevsky a sense that he occupied a special place in his cosmos, that his seizures held a grander purpose. Chico's visions, too, gave him a sense of purpose. His visions granted him a special place at his church, a position rare for a teenage labourer.

When we arrived on the third floor of the Hospital del Niño, Chico was lying on his side on the operating table. Our goal was to remove the grape-sized hamartoma and the source of the electricity causing his seizures. The cast and crew assembled was similar to my team back in LA, as were the names of the instruments, but some modern tools that had become so familiar to me were missing. Taking their place were a few others I'd read about only in accounts of the original pioneers of brain surgery.

All the plastic was gone. All those drapes, sheets and items that, in the US, are enclosed in plastic for individual use were brought out lovingly, wrapped in cloth like a newborn. The surgical-steel tools were smooth and weathered from decades of use. Some of the metal had been worn by the ergonomics of the surgeon's hand at the grips, like marble steps bevelled by millennia of tread, like boulders polished by river flow.

As junior surgeon, the job of opening the skull fell to me. The horseshoe incision over Chico's ear was a quick slice and the scalp slid apart, but the skull work over his temporal lobe was tricky. Just above the ear, the skull is very thin and, higher up, towards the top of the head, it's thicker. It's like the difference between a crêpe and a thick pancake, so you have to keep in mind the depth of the shell during the drilling. Jorge mentioned that making holes in the skull used to be an ancient spiritual ritual. 'Some patients want holes made, to let the demons out, they say, but we don't do that any more.' This practice, trephination, dating back thousands of years, found its most expert practitioners in the indigenous Chimú people, who used specialized tools and lived not far from where we were standing, in neighbouring Peru.

Making a hole in the skull is laborious even with an electric or a pneumatic drill. To make a hole in Chico's skull, I was using a hand drill called a Hudson Brace. I'd never held one before. A Hudson Brace has a ball on one end and a U-shaped bend in the middle that you crank to turn the bit. This surgical instrument had been used for hundreds of years to breach the skull. The one I was using looked very similar to an ornate version designed by sixteenth-century surgeon Giovanni Andrea della Croce and shown in his book *Chirurgiae Libri Septem*. Another illustration in this volume shows a nobleman lying in bed in his home, having a trephination performed on him. We were a long way from the Renaissance, but what I was doing was identical to what the surgeon in that illustration was doing over four hundred years ago – drilling a hole above the temporal lobe using a hand tool.

I made four large holes, and then Jorge used delicate chisels to finish lifting the circular bone the size of a biscuit from the skull. Unlike the pneumatic drill I used back home, there was less bone dust, meaning the bone cap fitted more snugly on the skull from which it was removed. I instantly thought of Karina and wondered whether chisels would have been better when I unroofed her spinal canal, whether my modern drill had had too much chatter and reverberation and had made the troughs just a few millimetres wider, allowing the roof of her spine to settle. Jorge was showing me how to do 'traditional' surgery. He kept his composure. I was thrown off by memories of Karina and grateful to have part of my face behind the mask so that my internal struggle wasn't visible. The surgery hadn't really even started yet.

For me, exposing the opalescent white naked flesh is always breathtaking. I love this part of brain surgery. I know I am witnessing something rare, something mysterious, something that comes with great responsibility. Entry into this world requires leaving distraction behind and displaying my craft.

Opening the dura, with the brain bulging underneath, means that the brain could get cut, too. Here, just a few millimetres too deep and a few thousand neurons disconnected could rob the patient of fundamental things like language and, possibly, spirituality. With Chico lying on his side under the canvas drapes that had become soft as Egyptian cotton from years of sterilization, we used the window over his left temporal lobe to cut and peel the dura in such a way that we could close it cleanly on our exit. We made an X-shaped cut in the dura – like 'X marks the spot'. The triangular leaflets folded back and the resultant square exposure of the brain looked like a mandala.

The dura was now out of the way, and a small tuft of misshapen tissue could be seen faintly in the shallow valleys of the sulci formed by the undulating ridges, or gyri. This was the hamartoma that we needed to remove. The human cortex forms just the outer one centimetre of our brain. Just as the rest of our brain is not homogeneous, the cortex has its own architecture, a cortical canopy like sedimentary layers of human evolution. Our modern brain is the neocortex. The paleocortex lies beneath it; from it we excavate our emotions. Our neocortex evolved from the paleocortex over thousands of years – glacially ballooning and pushing our foreheads forward. Its six vertical layers are responsible for sensory perception and spatial reasoning, motor commands, language and conscious thought.

Chico's hamartoma was an overgrowth that had upset this intricate topography, triggering 'aberrant' electricity that not only caused partial seizures but brought meaning, understanding and a connection to something profound to his life. Once quarantined to a single part of his brain, the aberrant electrical signals had now spread. They resonated globally across the hemispheres of his brain, and the seizures no longer delivered the divine to Chico's inner world but dropped him, unconscious, on the floor. Now, he had only one option – to have faith in us.

Epilepsy was not treated surgically until the 1930s, when the neurosurgeon Wilder Penfield developed what became known as the Montreal Procedure. It got the name because he was working at the Royal Victoria and Montreal General Hospital at the time. After removing the skull cap and exposing the brain under local anaesthetic, Penfield touched different parts of the brain with a small electrode. The patients were awake during surgery. Because the brain itself has no nerves, the mild electrical current could not cause them any pain. Because they were awake, patients could report what they were experiencing. Penfield realized that if he could find the spot on the brain that triggered the smell, sight or feeling that preceded an epileptic seizure, he could remove that tissue and potentially stop the seizures. Penfield would systematically map a patient's brain until he reached the source of the seizures and the patient announced, as one named Jean did, 'I have a funny feeling. It feels like an attack.' Another touch of the electrode on the same spot, and Jean said she heard people shouting at her. Still another, and she said, 'I feel like something dreadful is going to happen . . . please don't leave me,' and started weeping. At that point, Jean was put under general anaesthetic and that small piece of her temporal lobe was removed.

Penfield's awake surgery provided much more than

treatment for epilepsy. It offered a window into what had been an opaque world, the functional workings of the brain. During these surgeries, patients recounted memories, dreams and emotions, smells and sensations. He mapped the location of each of these, and more. The neurosurgeon told a story of testing a woman's brain with an electrode when she heard a melody. He touched the spot again, and she heard the melody again. He was so surprised he touched the spot thirty times. Each time, she heard the same melody.

By the mid-1950s, Penfield and his colleagues had performed more than a thousand surgeries for neurological disorders. Penfield and his patients were collaborators in this surreal exploration of the brain. Describing his relationship with his patients, Penfield said that although the surgeon 'commands the means and paraphernalia of science . . . the man who lies on the operating table beneath the sheet also listens and wonders and tries to understand. Between these two lie the secrets of the function of the brain.'

Penfield had provided the brain's Rosetta stone. Before him, we relied on fragments of information from injured brains, deducing brain function from what had been lost in the injury. Now the brain could speak its mind. With the electrode's mild electrical stimulation, Penfield was also able to produce otherworldly experiences. A thirty-three-year-old man with seizures who received electrical stimulation on his right temporal lobe, near his insula, cried out, 'Oh

God! I am leaving my body.' In other patients, Penfield elicited spiritual feelings by manipulating their temporal lobes. Penfield mapped the functions of different parts of the brain that had up to that point mostly been a source of mystery, a *terra incognita*. 'I am an explorer,' he said. 'But unlike my predecessors, who used compasses and canoes to discover unknown lands, I used a scalpel and a small electrode to explore and map the human brain.'

Before we removed Chico's hamartoma, we needed to follow in Penfield's footsteps and map the teenager's brain. Functional maps of the brain are accurate to the neighbourhood level, but for this work we searched for the address. We needed to be careful where we cut into Chico's temporal lobe. Not only belief but also language is located in the temporal lobe. We didn't want to injure a critical part of Chico's brain and take away his ability to utter or understand language.

Specific brain areas that control function are called 'eloquent'. Mapping the surface of Chico's brain allowed us to distinguish eloquent or non-eloquent areas in his cortical canopy. Once we had them separated, we knew where we could part the cortex to get to the deeper location of the hamartoma. Awake brain mapping is the standard of care for operating on the left temporal lobe. It shows you where it is safe to cut. Performing such a procedure when the patient is not awake would be reckless, like flying blind in the mountainous terrain of their humanity.

With Chico's hamartoma unconcealed, Jorge held a pen that delivered a gentle electric current to the teenager's brain. The tool was an extension of Jorge's hand, as if the nerves went from his fingertips into the metal instrument, reaching out to something beyond. He moved deftly, methodically, four decades of experience guiding him. I was enthralled. I was assisting someone who came from the generation that had followed Penfield, and he was now schooling me. On the surface of Chico's brain, Jorge marched and mapped. The gentle current led to activation and also suppression. At times, Chico talked. Other times, he stopped talking, something called speech arrest. If we cut at that spot, we'd be arresting his speech permanently.

Penfield placed small, numbered squares of paper in the patient's brain as he mapped it. We used small, colourful circles of paper that looked like they'd been made with a hole punch. A nurse had marked some with an X; others were left blank. Where electrical stimulation did not lead to speech arrest, an X-labelled circle was placed with forceps on the surface, like a pirate map showing where the treasure lay. That meant we could make a hole, a portal, through that part of the cortex. Thoughts and ability sprout from the cortex, and once past the cortex through a safe window, there is more latitude.

During the mapping, Chico would at times count and read normally. And then, on occasion, with a cadence that was almost musical, he would speak like someone reciting the words of a song or a poem. Words flowed from his mouth: *arboles, animales, Dios, rios, madre, juntos, siempre*. Trees, animals, God, rivers, mother, together, always. Those were the words I recall clearly.

During the surgery, when we mapped and tickled the surface of the brain with the electrode, it evoked the same feelings in Chico as his seizures did. This surgical provocation, with Chico awake, would offer him one last connection to his most cherished thoughts and emotions. It was the last time he would experience that depth of spirituality. As he talked of God and nature, I wanted to ask Jorge if Chico was unique, or if the connection he felt with the divine was typical among his epilepsy patients.

Jorge could sense that I wanted to ask this question and said, '*Es comun*,' it's common, before I asked. Do these awake patients often speak of nature and heaven? The ones that are Catholic sometimes speak of Christ, Jorge said. The children from the tribes usually speak of both, since they have a mixture of faiths, feelings, understandings, experiences.

As we rounded off the surgery, Jorge said, 'I hope he accepts his next life.'

Sadly, the words and feelings that Chico uttered during the surgery would be the last of his deep connection with his personal spirituality. It was the 'side effect' of curing him of epilepsy. He woke up and moved on with his life, able to work again without seizures, but he never regained the spiritual connection that was so special to him.

Over dinner at his home, Jorge's wife mentioned that there are 'undiscovered' tribes in the Amazon, tribes that have never been exposed to any outside human contact or religion, who think high-flying planes are UFOs. To them, they are. Jorge and I looked at each other and, with the residue of that morning in our minds, he said, '*Me pregunto qué dirían si mapeamos los misterios de su mente.*' 'I wonder what they would speak of if we could map the mysteries of their minds.'

Listening to Chico during his awake brain surgery made me appreciate that belief is probably more than culture and upbringing. It has a mysterious physical presence in the brain. I also know, as a scientist, that belief activates physiology that helps my patients endure the stress of surgery and avoid the despair of a deadly disease.

But if there are parts of the brain associated with religious feeling, does this mean faith is innate or acquired, or both? Even today, this most essential question remains a mystery. Over the years, I've watched my patients turn to their beliefs for solace during their most trying times. Before surgery, many have asked me to join them in a moment of prayer or reflection, and I am honoured to be included. The strength and meaning belief can provide is undeniable.

6.

Threat

The patient was a mother in her thirties, with kids, and a manageable tumour. If we removed it all, she would be cured, but that was difficult. It was better to leave behind a little tumour, and still significantly extend her life, than risk profound injury by being too aggressive. In a case like hers, most senior surgeons could get most, if not all, of her tumour and not injure the patient.

I was a neurosurgery resident, a brain surgeon in training, and I'd scrubbed in for a case with the professor of the department, who was about to make a mistake that would ruin this person. The woman's skull was open, the forehead bone removed, and both frontal lobes were exposed. The professor and I were standing on either side of the patient, sharing a surgical microscope with eyepieces directly opposite each other. It's like two people using the same set of binoculars. Our hands were outside the patient, but our instruments were about eight inches deep in the brain, so deep the broad spray of light in the operating theatre failed to shine into the small area where we were working. Instead, we relied on an intensely bright light shining straight down from the microscope. In this illuminated area we would need to perform several hundred steps, using delicate instruments under high magnification.

For hours, we spread, pruned and dissected inside natural valleys of brain tissue, working our way deeper into the patient's brain to get to the tumour. As I worked, the professor watched and assisted. Many of the arteries and veins in the brain have names. Many do not. A vital part of the seven years of neurosurgery training is learning the rare vessel that can be sacrificed and which ones need to be preserved, which ones can be cut safely and which ones can't. You won't find this information in *Anatomy 101*. Even physicians who aren't brain surgeons don't know the terms. It's not taught until you are in the trade. The brain is such a unique and convoluted structure, the neck, chest and abdomen look basic by comparison.

I reached a branch off the main trunk of the anterior cerebral artery, which delivers blood to the front and centre of the brain. This particular branch tricks novices into thinking it is something that can be divided. It isn't. It's the recurrent artery of Heubner, so infamous in neurosurgery it's hammered into residents from day one. The artery is called recurrent because it breaks off the main trunk and loops backwards like a hairpin turn on the Formula 1 course in

Monaco. It's infamous because it supplies blood to unique structures in the brain. Damaging it can harm a patient in a bizarre constellation of ways.

When you're performing surgery inside a living person, anatomy does not look like a picture in a textbook. You get only glimpses, often obscured by blood and fatigue. The recurrent artery of Heubner resembles a backward-turning knuckle. It is the red wire that needs to be avoided at all costs. I saw it. The professor must have seen it. I dissected the gossamer fibres of brain tissues so the two of us could see it better, know it was there and leave it alone. Better to identify and expose the recurrent artery of Heubner than have it lurking somewhere, unseen or partially hidden. That's when it happened: I saw the tips of the microscissors come into my field of view under the microscope.

When the professor called for the scissors, I thought he was anticipating a manoeuvre where I needed him to cut. There was no need for them, not yet, but the scissors were there and moving into the highly magnified and brightly illuminated area where I was working. It was like someone placing their hand in front of an old-fashioned movie projector. The professor and I were face to face, inches apart, separated by the microscope. No one else in the operating room could see what was happening inside the patient's brain as the professor's scissors moved towards the artery.

'Sir, Heubner,' I whispered, without looking up from the microscope. That warning should have been enough. The blades of his scissors advanced. It was like watching the shark in *Jaws* closing in. 'Sir, Heubner,' I repeated, more urgently. He was about to injure the artery. The results would be devastating for the patient. Hitting the artery would mean that this young mother would have a weak left leg. Her crotch would also be numb for the rest of her life, and what would happen to her mind would be far worse. She would be abulic, meaning she would have an inability to act decisively. There would be a slowness about how she engaged with the world. She would be apathetic, uninterested, inert, laconic, inactive.

What should I do? What could I do? I was only a trainee, a neurosurgery resident, a twenty-nine-year-old grunt, three years into my training, working 120 hours a week. I was married with two young sons, aged four and one. The professor was everyone's boss, and we were trained to 'trust the professor'. Be a good boy. There is a saying in neurosurgery: 'It takes a real man to be a boy this long.' He was the professor. His power was absolute. Not long before, he had summarily fired a surgeon with a pregnant spouse. No warning. At the end of the seven years, the professor's word, and his word alone, would determine whether I was deemed qualified to join the ranks of practising surgeons. Showing up the professor in the operating theatre was a good way to get fired.

And what if it wasn't Heubner? What if I was wrong? What if the artery was harmless? What if cutting it was inconsequential? I wanted to be wrong. I wanted the professor to be right. That would make what was about to happen so much easier. But I knew that what we were looking at under our shared microscope was Heubner. I also knew I might lose my job by stopping him.

As the professor's scissors bore down on the artery, my choices were stark. Do nothing, and this patient's life would be wrecked. The error would be written off, the terrible outcome explained away as the result of unforeseeable complications caused by 'unusual anatomy' or 'patient disease'. These vague phrases would serve as a pardon at the weekly Morbidity and Mortality (M&M) meeting. The professor would meet with the patient and her family. His title would go a long way to absolving him in their eyes. My career would be unscathed.

Do something, and my career as a neurosurgeon would almost certainly be over. The professor would probably kick me out of neurosurgery, and I'd need to begin training in a new field. I would be starting over in emergency medicine or anaesthesia or general medicine, specialties I would find less interesting, less important, less challenging. I liked brain surgery. I liked the danger of it. I loved how it demanded my peak attention and performance. I'd started my residency in general surgery with the intention of becoming a heart surgeon. I joined the neurosurgery programme when the professor fired someone who had the highest scores in the country, leaving a vacancy. I was a battlefield pick-up. Once I was in neurosurgery, I never looked back. Neurosurgery was where I wanted to be.

Thoughts flooded my brain as the scissors closed in on the recurrent artery of Heubner, and then one rose to the top: Fuck it. Both options – acting and not acting – were terrible, but I wouldn't be able to live with myself if I let him devastate this woman's life. Now that I'd decided to stop him, what could I do? We were moments from catastrophe. I thought about looking up from my highly magnified view of the woman's brain and physically reaching out to stop his hand from going any further. I didn't have time. The scissors were advancing fast.

At the last second I diverted the metal suction in my left hand and the drinking-straw-like tube blocked the professor's scissor blades. I could feel the scissors closing in on my metal instrument and then the gentle reverberations; it was as though I had snared a small fish. He knew he had become disoriented and that I had stopped a catastrophic error, but no one showed up the professor. The prospect of saying goodbye to my future hit me in the gut.

'You're done,' the professor said. The implications were endless, and all of them were bad. Done with this operation? Done with this year of training? Done with neurosurgery? Done ever working in an American hospital? That's the kind of power he had, and I had every reason to expect my fate would involve one or more of these sickening options.

No one else in the operating room had witnessed what had happened under the microscope. There was no one to testify on my behalf. What had happened was between the two of us. The professor and I stopped working and looked up. Our eyes met to the side of the microscope's binoculars. His face was expressionless, but his eyes reeked of disdain.

'Finish the case,' he said, and I did so, doing my best to focus on the immediate work and not on my uncertain future while he watched on.

Before he left the room, as I was putting in the finishing sutures, he said, 'No need to round on the patient.' Rounding is checking on patients after surgery, answering questions from patients and family members. It's something surgeons typically hate. For someone like the professor, one of the perks of being a senior surgeon at a teaching hospital is that residents usually do the rounding and other post-operative work such as making notes, pulling drains and writing discharge instructions. Asking me not to round was highly unusual, but in this case he wanted to control the narrative, not only for the patient and her family, but for me.

An hour later, as was customary, the professor broke scrub, ripping off his gown and gloves, and went to the phone to dictate the details of the operation for the patient's medical records and billing. Like all surgeons, he dictated rapid fire, sounding like a Texas auctioneer selling cattle but with a New York accent. At the end of the dictation, I heard him say, 'I performed the operation skin to skin.' That customary lie allowed the professor, as senior surgeon, to collect the most surgical fees. 'Skin to skin' is where the senior surgeon performs the entire operation, from initial incision to the final closing stitch. In teaching hospitals, this is unusual. The bulk of many operations are typically turned over to inexperienced hands, surgeons in training.

When I started surgical training, I was surprised to find that some practising surgeons were inept. Given the major advances in surgery, I anticipated an elite corps of the technically capable. My credulity was punctured quickly by reality. The surgeons I encountered were all too human. Their skills varied and often had nothing to do with intelligence. When surgeons made mistakes, which was alarmingly often, they'd wind up presenting at the surgeons-only M&M meeting.

By showing up the professor in surgery, I had avoided the kind of terrible mistake that would have landed me in front of M&M, standing in front of my peers presenting on a woman whose recurrent artery of Heubner had been cut. Still, preventing a catastrophe in the operating theatre had had the perverse effect of putting my job and my career at risk. The professor was powerful. His ego was bruised. I was now aware of his potentially dangerous surgical abilities, and he knew it. But the professor wasn't done with me. He would test me, just not in the way I expected.

By this point in my life, threat was familiar to me. A decade earlier, in my late-teenage years, I had faced another kind of threat, a smouldering malevolence next door to my home that eventually erupted in violence. That experience had given me some armour, a way to manage the professor.

The houses in my neighbourhood were small and L-shaped, strange mirror images, chiral, almost like your hands, which look identical but can't fit into the same glove. The open face of the Ls faced each other and the doors and walkways were ten strides apart. There was no avoiding your neighbours. The family next door to us was a woman and her three sons. Larry was closest to my age, but still ten years older.

Larry's mother would give me, the kid next door, five dollars to mow their small lawn with a push mower, or a dollar to bring in her groceries for her. Back then, they were very generous sums. I never asked to be paid. She insisted. I can't imagine the stress of raising those three boys alone. I never saw any sign of it. She was always kind to me and I felt a loving, accepting and nurturing vibe from her, which made what happened later with Larry even more disconcerting. By the time all that went down, though, she had already passed away.

Even before I headed to the University of California, Berkeley, Larry had started trying out his slowly blossoming street philosophy of the ignored and imposed upon, the aggrieved majority being cheated out of their rightful dominion. 'If they can say black power, why can't we say white pride?' he wanted to know. He hadn't yet taken the next fateful step. He wasn't talking about white power. Not yet.

When I decided to drop out of college and return to the old neighbourhood, Larry was still there. His mother had died recently, of cancer. He had been let go from work, his perspective on those around him had changed. He felt disenfranchised, someone whose hold on the middle class was slipping away, and I could see it from his point of view. I was still a teenager, but I was sympathetic. When he lost his job, he felt as if it had been taken from him because immigrants were undercutting him. It became tribal, and in his eyes I was part of the enemy tribe.

He was being left behind. His only outlet was a garage gym, and he invested more and more effort into working out. Steroids and ''roid rage' came into the mix, and something more. The year I returned home, something had changed, and he wasn't shy about it. Against the far wall of the garage there was a flag with a Nazi swastika at its dark heart. Visible but still semi-concealed, as if he was testing out his new identity.

As people moved on or moved out or lost interest, Larry's resentment and frustration grew, and morphed into disgust. Disgust turned to hate. The feeling became mutual. And then it became a weird power struggle. If I was apologetic for no reason, he would smell blood, and it would fall even harder on me. If I initiated aggression, I would be playing into his hands: he would get what he wanted.

I'd see Larry sometimes, when I was trying to slip in and out of my home. When he walked away, he did it with purpose, a shot across the bow, what some felons call 'back arms'. Back arms are triceps, the three heads of the muscles extending from the shoulder to the forearm forming a perfect vertical canvas for his first tattoo, a dual billboard in an old-English font: WHITE. PRIDE. He had a strange physicality: Arnold Schwarzenegger mixed with something ugly – Charles Manson, maybe.

When I moved back, I personified what Larry now resented most. His mission became single-minded: to dominate. Stage one was verbal warfare, and he embraced this with gusto. It was as if I represented a whole range of brown. The filth that came out of his mouth was long and varied: redskin, spick, sand-nigger, wetback. I was strangely intrigued by the breadth of racial terminology he had and how I had come to embody such a wide range of humanity.

Larry's goal was to have me tap out, a psychological surrender, like submitting in a mixed martial arts fight. That parachute cord was not one he would later offer me. He wanted to see defeat and fear in my eyes, and only then would he relent. His verbal assaults mounted and they weighed on me from the moment I woke up in the morning until the moment I went to sleep. Still, I refused to give him any outward sign that he was getting to me. My only power was in showing no sign of intimidation. The walk from the street to the front door became a test of both my mettle and the strategy I had devised to endure the verbal onslaught.

As the predictable vitriol rained down on me as I walked to my front door, I would pause for five seconds to face the torrent. Let it hail. Let it pummel. Bathe in it a bit. But my face would be blank, emotionless. I wanted my reaction to confuse Larry, and I wanted this confusion to gnaw at him. After this pause, I would resume my walk to the door.

I might not have come home at all, but my mother was there, recuperating from chemotherapy and a cancer diagnosis. She spent her time in her room, a bucket next to her side of the bed in case she needed to throw up. I'd leave crackers and water on her nightstand as she did her best to defy her fate. I'd be in the living room of our small home, at war with a different foe. I understood that Larry was going to raise the stakes. I knew he would escalate, but I had no idea how.

Living under the weight of threat, I became

vigilant. I just didn't know what to do. The threat was episodic, existential, never-ending. Sometimes I felt I was overreacting; sometimes, underreacting. All the while, he and I would do the polite thing and keep our warfare mostly out of sight of my mother. I was becoming a stranger to myself, an unfamiliar animal. Tender and loyal to my loved ones, but on edge and tactical as I prepared for the unforeseeable.

Bracing myself for the verbal lashing from Larry guided my behaviour. I felt surprisingly in control, despite the hail of sensations, emotions and thoughts. Faced with a threat, people often describe the situation as 'fight or flight', but it is more nuanced than that. Sometimes one doesn't engage or flee; sometimes, you brace.

We are all injury averse. When I say 'we', even single-cell organisms will drift away from noxious stimuli. The moment there is life, there is threat, and the most basic form of behaviour in animals is a reflex, an automatic response to a stimulus. Think of when a general practitioner taps the tendon below your kneecap and your leg kicks forward: that is reflex. It can't be trained or thought away – the neuro-anatomical pathway is just in your spinal cord and doesn't even reach the brain. As we go through life, our brains are constantly sprouting and pruning branches between neurons based on what we learn about the world. As we experience what is sharp, or hot, or painful, we learn to avoid them. Sometimes, however, we need to countermand these basic impulses. Sometimes, we need to move towards the threat and accept the pain to get past it.

'Fight or flight' is not a switch that goes on or off without your directive; your thinking and your emotional brain first need to assess the threat as real. In a part of the brain so ancient we share it with non-mammalian ancestors, you'll find the pons. The pons is the widest part of the brainstem and it manufactures and releases its own adrenaline into the brain and body. This is the same chemical we inject as a last-ditch effort when a patient's blood pressure collapses.

A tiny, paired cluster of cells in your pons, left and right, synthesize their adrenaline. These cells comprise less than 1 per cent of your brain's cellular landscape, but they synthesize and spray this intensely potent chemical. Adrenaline docks on cellular ports across your arteries, gut and heart, and the response is always one way. Vessels shuttle more blood to muscles, the gut gets less blood, the heart beats faster and stronger. Only one part of us remains independent from this chemical that is so ancient it's found in jellyfish: the brain.

Whether you're pursued in a back alley or watching a scary movie from the safety of the living-room couch, the pons releases the same adrenaline. The brain assesses the true risk. Adrenaline is contextualized before we react – before we change our behaviour in response. Early in the twentieth century, the Spanish physician Gregorio Marañón demonstrated this by injecting patients with adrenaline. Because they weren't in danger, they didn't have the 'fight or flight' impulse. They experienced the fast-beating heart associated with a dangerous situation, but not the fear. The dual nature of our experience makes us human. Our emotional brain may not be able to read out the context, but our thinking mind is never completely separated from these instincts. Watching a horror movie, our heart may beat faster, but we don't flee when the chainsaw-wielding killer leaps out of the wardrobe. We know the adrenaline is permitted – we even welcome it.

One day, positioned at the window, I saw two cars roll up as I peeked under the curtain. They were not two random cars that just happened to be driving up the street at the same time, they were in a strange formation. These two cars were being driven by people in cahoots, I could feel it. The cars coursed past the houses and turned left at the next block. One of them was Larry's Bronco. Why would Larry drive past his own house? I knew. He was planting his accomplice's getaway car and swinging back. Darkness at noon.

A man appeared at our front door. He had a tattoo on his face. Back then, having tattoos typically signified that you were a biker or a criminal. A teardrop below the outer edge of your eye signified that you were a convict, that you had been in prison. This man had one. I was six feet tall and weighed twelve and a half stone. He probably had two inches and two and a half stone on me.

Larry had hired a goon to come at my family and me, probably for fifty dollars. With Larry standing behind him, the hired muscle knocked and knocked, banged and banged. I stood with my back to the inside wall that separated the main front window and the wooden front door. The house rattled. I worried they were going to kick in the door. And as I heard my mother ask what was happening, I could hear the depletion in her voice. Larry had me in a jam. I could not let my mother bear the weight of her cancer and now this crisis. I needed to go out there and eat some pain, the way she had been absorbing the pain of her cancer.

I stepped outside. They descended.

At that point, in my mind, it was still a fair fight. The blows were bearable, startling, but familiar and endurable, like tumbling off a bike. I was navigating a crash. 'How long could this go on, in daylight?' I felt myself starting to think.

Then the felon connected with brass knuckles and I felt a pain like a lightning bolt discharge on my left side. It felt as if a red-hot wire clothes hanger had been pressed up inside my back and the side of my chest. It was an electric pain, unlike anything I had felt before. Not the raw pain of a broken leg, or the sharp pain of a cut, this was purely electric, as though

I'd been bitten by an electric eel. The strike cracked two ribs.

Our ribcage, as a whole, provides a shield for the organs behind it, but each rib individually is a dry branch, and snappable if struck just right. Ribs are thin enough to be cut during surgery by a device that looks like large nail clippers. The nerves run only on the underside of each human rib. The ribcage makes a good shield, porous unlike the skull, and flexible, which allows the lungs to fill. The ribcage can return to its original form after stress and deformation – the engineering definition of resilience.

I realized I was OK under the flurry and purpose was a balm to the screaming pain in my side. This was so much more than 'fight or flight'. I wasn't feeling fear or panic. I felt hate and anger.

My brain finally allowed adrenaline to release its potential in a surge of revolt. I retaliated. By now, cars had stopped on the usually quiet side street. Larry called a stop to it, and the felon ran off to the getaway car he'd stashed around the corner. Larry and I glared at each other one last time. Neighbours. I watched on one knee, defiant as he receded into his garage.

I took a drink from the garden hose that was lying near me, wiped my face, unlocked the door and slid inside the house. Standing up to hit the deadbolt was the last painful effort I made. I sat on the floor next to the living-room sofa, next to a knife I'd planted there but forgotten to take outside with me.

Every breath made me want to groan. There, on the floor of my parents' house, I felt the surge of hormones, a flood of chemicals coursing through me. Taming adrenaline that has been given purpose is not quick or easy. It was like trying to chill after a car crash.

Sitting there on the floor with my back to the front door, I could smell the residue of smoke from the convict. Like it was date night for him. But that smoke wasn't cigarettes, it was something more *Breaking Bad*, more cooked up. It was a chemical smoke, like a burning plastic factory. Crystal meth. He'd gotten jacked up to battle. I remember that smell vividly, even now, three decades later.

It should come as no surprise that the part of our brain that processes smell, the olfactory lobe, is directly connected to the hippocampus, which is shaped like a pair of seahorses, inside each temple in front of our ears, and is responsible for constructing short- and long-term memories. That's why a certain smell can trigger such a powerful emotional memory. Sight, touch, taste and sound do not have this literal connection to the seat of emotion and memory.

Odour-evoked memory has been dubbed the 'Proust phenomenon' because of the writer Marcel Proust's famous description of being transported to a long-forgotten moment in his childhood by the smell of a madeleine dipped in linden tea. Not all odour-induced memories are positive. The felon's smell is singed in my memory, and my frontal lobes can't erase that, however hard I try. Despite all our neural and cognitive horsepower, some visceral mind imprints are indelible.

We don't always get to choose to avoid the threats we face in life, nor are all threats the same. If a driver veers into our lane, the threat is immediate. If we are diagnosed with cancer, as my mother was, the threat persists. With Larry, the threat was somewhere in between. I knew his aim was to humiliate me, and the months of mind warfare between us had weighed on me constantly, no matter how hard I tried to present an implacable face to Larry.

Every day brought a firestorm of thoughts and feelings. There was no Hollywood ending to my story with Larry. No tale of revenge to tell. In the coming months, he sold his mother's house and moved away. We stood our ground. The following year, rumours circulated among our neighbours that he was doing time in prison.

Years later, right after my confrontation with the professor, I drove to my home, my career threatened, my future obscured. I'd been allowed briefly into the club, into the elite fellowship of neurosurgery, and now it looked like I was getting kicked out, expelled for not knowing my place, for not showing blind loyalty. Even worse, the professor had the power to hold my family's livelihood as a weapon against me. The threat this time was not some hired thug, but a powerful surgeon, a professor and my boss.

At that point, I had no idea what was going to happen. But as with my experience with Larry, I had to find a way to move on with my life. How I chose to do that – how we all choose to cope – determines whether we will crack under the weight of threat or bounce back from it. Fortunately, evolution and experience has equipped us to deal with adversity.

Our ancestors, from the distant past right up to our parents, have endowed us with armour. It is also something we can build up throughout our lives. We are adaptive to the widest range of environments possible and to the widest number of threats possible. The adaptation is one that has to be developed and then deployed situationally. This has been called a stress-inoculating effect. The popular word for it these days is resilience. Engineers might see this as the ability to become altered under stress and return to the original form. When it comes to the mind, though, resilience is more than responding to a threat and reverting to a prior state. The mind is altered, changed, reconfigured into a more fortified version of itself.

The brain is always changing, and we have the power to steer it, to take advantage of it. My patients after brain surgery can recover lost function, so you shouldn't doubt that our healthy brains can manage our relationship to threat. This is all down to plasticity of thinking. What determines how we react, our behaviour and how we cope is not 'hard-wired'. There are no 'wires'. There are no 'circuits'. But there are assemblies and ensembles of neurons. And opportunities. What if we could trim or loosen the sails on what we want to accept, accommodate, integrate from our challenges? The strategy we choose to cope with a threat is everything. Actively facing our fears, problem solving and seeking the support of others is a path to resilience from the immediate threat. It also helps produce long-term resilience. The alternative is what's been dubbed passive coping: denial, avoidance and disengaging.

Resilience means sublimating a threat by putting the stress it generates to use. The resilience you carry and demonstrate when faced with a new crisis is one type of resilience – systemic resilience, meaning you have it within you. I've seen this type of resilience first hand in patients who have gone through trauma, assault, cancer and have maintained their psychological well-being rather than spinning into disarray. I'm inspired by them, and use their journeys to inform myself and others.

If threat plunges you into maladaptive and self-destructive holes, the story of your resilience is not yet written. If you have been knocked off your foundation, that doesn't mean you aren't resilient. With time, you can allow internal processing to germinate a new perspective, something called processive resilience. Resilience is both what you've built up and what you *will* build up – what you bring to the fight and what the fight brings out in you. That way, you can embrace your journey from the individual perspective of your struggle, your endurance, your triumph – all from inside your interior life, where it matters most.

Some hits are so punishing that just enduring them is true resilience. Other hits sink in, take hold and force you to purge them out. You don't want unproductive thoughts and emotions that are poured out under threat to cement into the emotional foundation of self. Going forward, you have the potential to showcase your resilience, not through what happened to you, but by how you recovered from it.

Few have to cope with a bigger threat than stage 4 cancer patients, who face something ominously but appropriately termed an 'existential threat'. They need to find a way to live, a mind frame, an approach with which to brace themselves for the results from tests and scans and the gripping concern any time something hurts. These are the minor symptoms most of us easily ignore but, for these patients, everything is tied to the question: could that be my cancer spreading? In between those moments, they somehow excavate the psychological and emotional reserve to live their lives.

People ask me if it isn't depressing to be a cancer surgeon. Why? I respond. My patients don't depress me. They enlighten me. They inspire me. They have developed the strength and the ability to experience joy with mortality teetering like an anvil over their heads. Most tell me they wish they had applied these strengths before they learned they had cancer. Why, they ask me, did quality of life become a priority for them only after a cancer diagnosis? Their crisis management has improved my quality of life – I've learned life lessons from cancer patients. For cancer patients, managing a threat doesn't render them helpless, and they don't have to learn optimism. For the most part, I don't see the 'learned helplessness' popularized by Ivan Pavlov and his dogs, or even Martin Seligman's 'learned optimism'. I see realism.

Cancer patients have shown me that most of life's experiences are double-edged. Hypervigilance is always painted as something excessive, but I suspect that many of us live under a threat that requires it. Responsibilities like the ones I have as a surgeon, and others have as, say, air-traffic controllers, require sustained focus, so vigilance needs to be cultivated. Hypervigilance can be of service.

For some of us, there is no escaping the threat of economic hardship or sexual or physical abuse. Some develop disabling psychological or health problems as a result, while others show resilient behaviour. The answer to these differences is not built into our DNA. Identical twins have the same DNA but can respond to the same threats very differently. If one develops stress-related depression, the other twin will develop stress-related depression only about 40 per cent of the time. This means that environment has played a role.

The difference, it turns out, is epigenetics, where

molecular alterations to DNA or proteins change how genes behave without actually changing the underlying DNA. Our genetic blueprint is so long it has to be wrapped around protein scrolls to stop it from tangling up. This design also serves to cordon off DNA, making it inaccessible, and thereby regulating our genetic code at the highest level. Hence the name *epigenetics*. It turns out that the unwinding of these scrolls is deeply influenced by our life experiences.

Sometimes, these epigenetic changes are damaging. Other times, they are fortifying. Either way, the life lessons and adaptations are passed on to our children. The strategies and manoeuvres by which we navigate crises are transmissible to our progeny without any change in our DNA. Heritability is not just based on the long, haphazard progress of DNA mutations but on epigenetic modifications passed directly to your descendants with changes in your sperm or egg. No need to wait to give advice to your offspring – build it into them. Epigenetic heritability creates an immediacy to your legacy and makes it a responsibility as well. To me, this is inspiring science within us. Jonas Salk, the discoverer of the first polio vaccine, was prescient when he said, 'I'm just trying to be a good ancestor.'

We all face threats in our lives: the threat of abuse, pain and loss. We can choose how to respond to them. I felt the only way to manage the threat that Larry posed was to take it head on and then try to grow from it and not let it turn into a series of intrusive thoughts and fears on loop. Thankfully, once it was over, he moved away, so I was able to process what had happened and move on myself.

Having been through that early in life, other threats did not seem as dire. Coping in a high-stress situation can improve our problem-solving abilities, perception and learning and prepare us for the next difficult or unpredictable situation. An adaptive psychological immunity. Having endured Larry's threat, I was better prepared to face the professor. When he threatened to end my career as a neurosurgeon, I knew I could get past it.

7.

Addiction

The computer screen flagged her as a self-referral, which meant she had somehow found me on her own. All the other patients that day were listed as consults, scheduled to see me because doctors had referred them. When she introduced herself to me, she said, '*Yo soy Puerto Riqueña, y una doctora.*' 'I am Puerto Rican, and a doctor.'

She was in a halo vest, a misleading name for a contraption that keeps your head connected to your neck. The name comes from the matte-black metal ring that appears to float around the forehead. Though it seems to be levitating, the ring is actually held in place with four screws that evenly pierce inward from the steel, puncturing the scalp and half the thickness of the skull. She was accompanied by her brother, father and sister, who from time to time would tenderly apply antibiotic ointment to the spots where the screws met the skin of her forehead. From this miserable crown of screws, four thin aluminium spokes jutted down to shoulder pads, two in front and two at the back.

La doctora was in a wheelchair because the halo was so top heavy, and sitting rigidly because she couldn't tilt her head up or down or pivot it left or right. I lowered myself to one knee so I could meet her gaze and show my respect. That restriction of movement was the whole point of the halo vest, because the bones at the base of her skull and the top of her spine were eaten up by cancer and could no longer bear the weight of her head. Any movement would snap the brittle bone that remained. It may have looked like incarceration and torture, but it was what she needed and the best that modern medicine could offer.

Puerto Rico is one of five inhabited American territories. Although the residents pay US taxes, the territories have a medical and surgical infrastructure far inferior to that on the mainland and Hawaii. All of them are limited in the care they can provide, although the health-care workers make the most of what they have. What this patient needed was far beyond what was possible in Puerto Rico. What she needed was only even theoretically possible at elite US cancer centres.

Surgeons in Miami, Washington, New York and Boston didn't want to take her case on. Now, she was in my clinic, ready to spend her life savings, to pay cash out of pocket, for me, the cast and crew, and for materials – as well as, the most costly of all, the hospital stay itself. In the United States, unless a procedure is covered by private insurance or one of the government health-care programmes, it's cash only.

As we spoke, her eyes were strong, but I could tell she was also braced for the next ungodly rip of pain that would strike her face and neck on the left. Nerves inside her were being devoured by cancer. As a physician, she knew that no surgery would cure her. Her quest, the reason she had travelled from surgeon to surgeon, hospital to hospital, was driven by a simple wish. She wanted to see her son graduate from college in six months' time. I think her father, sister and brother were really there to indulge her, to help her buy hope, although there was next to none.

Her uterine cancer had spread, making it stage 4, but she was in an unusual category of advanced cancer where it exists only in one spot outside its origin. Many stage 4 cancer patients have lots of cancer spread – often the body becomes riddled with it; this is called disseminated metastases. These patients are systemically sick and often their awareness is also diminished. But *la doctora* was wide awake, wearing a halo and waiting to be eaten alive from one particular spot in her body – the base of her skull, behind her left ear lobe. Without surgery, she would simply have to wait for the cancer to do its dastardly deed, to burrow into the brainstem, the part of the brain responsible for such basic functions as breathing, heart rate and consciousness.

No medicine or radiation options were left. Those options had been exhausted, as was the patient. The screw on her left forehead had pinned her scalp up a bit, giving her face a weird one-eyebrow-raised expression – like the late Sean Connery's James Bond. Her eyes were strong in their sockets, though, and then she made this plea: 'Cut it out of me. I can suffer the pain, but only because I hope to see my son graduate.' The possibility of surgery gave her hope, and hope was her strength. Hope was her heroin. In front of me lay a new surgery that prominent East Coast hospitals had said was impossible. Leaders in the field had said that her cancer was inoperable, that no one could remove the cancer without losing the patient. The challenge was my stimulant.

After Karina's surgery, I had become addicted to taking on the nearly impossible, as if this would somehow set things right. That drove me for years. Doing extremely difficult surgeries was my gateway drug. Over time, my skills rose to the point where I was considered capable, talented even. As I improved, my addiction metamorphosed. I was no longer secretly being driven by righting a wrong but by the thrill that came with defeating other surgeons in our own Olympics of sorts. Then I shifted one gear higher. I wanted not just to be better than other surgeons, faster, with smaller incisions and fewer complications, but to work on cases they couldn't do: the 'big whacks'. A 'big whack' is the phrase we use for an extensive operation that few surgeons can handle. It's a term I would later find repulsive.

Narcissism became a driver to achieve, and I was a narcissist with a chip on my shoulder. I was antagonistic, adversarial almost to a fault. I was hyperacute, but only to criticisms, not to praise.

I used perceived past grievances and grudges to fuel my ambition. Maybe it was the look in those students' eyes when I dropped out of Berkeley and began working in the cafeteria. Maybe it was the looks from the locals when I was growing up, thinking I wasn't tough enough. I didn't want to care about what they thought. That's what I tried to tell myself. That's what my English teacher at Compton Community College in South Central LA told me after I'd re-enrolled in college. Mr Jett was a mentor who taught with passion and purpose. His mantra was: 'What other people think about you is none of your business.' I tried to hold on to his words when I was feeling reactive to slights, real or perceived, and I saw slights everywhere.

Offence turned to resentment turned to competition – surgery became the place where I could assert my *self*, my ego, and relish the victory. But no victory was enough, and I was hooked on the challenge. To be the first one to invent an operation that was nearly impossible for other surgeons. I can't tell when I temporarily lost my emotional compass, the moment where the needle moved from doing surgery for the patients to doing it for myself. Fortunately, our interests were aligned. Serve my patients and feed my ego. Feed my ego and serve my patients.

But addiction, no matter what the end result, is unhealthy, a monkey on your back, a physical or mental dependence that commandeers the pleasure and pain centres of your brain. Mine were hijacked by this overwhelming urge to do what no other surgeon had done. There is a deep competition among talented surgeons, so when I did perform something no one else had, the high lasted for months. This in turn gave me more opportunities, because the case would be published in medical journals, and entire neurosurgical societies would hear about it. If I pulled off this surgery, the surgical literature and conferences would showcase my work. Unfamiliar. Fresh. Creative.

Although she wasn't a surgeon, *la doctora* was a physician. She understood the gravity of the location of her cancer. She knew that the malignant seeds from her uterus had taken root on tenuous soil. Her surgery had a high chance of intra-operative death. Initially, I said I wouldn't do it. I didn't see any upside for this patient, no matter my private attraction to taking on the challenge. So, she asked again, can you cut it out of me? She asked me what the chances were that I could remove the tumour nestled between her brain and her spinal cord – even though it would inevitably come back months later – without her dying in surgery or immediately afterwards from the injuries sustained in surgery.

I told her there was a 90 per cent chance we couldn't

get it out without hurting her in a way that would be, for most, worse than death.

She said, 'Then you have answered my prayers, because if no one tries, then the chance this cancer tortures and maims me is 100 per cent.' I hadn't seen it that way, but I appreciated my patient's perspective.

When I'd taken part in the hemicorpectomy, when half the patient's body was removed, I'd wondered if the patient's focus on the 10 per cent chance of a cure was misguided. He had other options. He could have gone with a less drastic approach that would probably have given him years, even if it wasn't a 'cure'. The irresistible allure of a cure made all of us lose sight of the likely disruption to his self. With *la doctora*, her options were suffering and more suffering. I was asked to alleviate pain and prevent disability; we both knew that my efforts wouldn't extend her life. Palliation would allow her to have one last cherished moment with her son. Or a death in the operating theatre where she went down fighting.

She knew there was little chance of success. Without surgery, her fate was sealed. Scheduling surgery would at least allow her to hope, and hope is therapeutic. Hope is a strange thing. It's a positive emotion that comes when things are dark, or at least uncertain. Hope is a true mixture of thought and emotion that usually arrives unbidden, a gift. A lot of surgeons are leery of hope, especially of offering patients false hope, but hope can be empowering. Hope requires agency, planning and energy in order to achieve a goal. Hopelessness brings a 'why bother?' paralysis, or worse. Expecting a bad result makes it more likely you will experience it, a self-fulfilling prophecy called the nocebo effect; it's the opposite of the placebo effect. *La doctora* sought me out to engineer hope in the bleak circumstances she was facing. Despite the odds, her plea was one I didn't deny.

If she hadn't been a physician, my answer might have been different – even given my desire to perform uniquely challenging surgeries. But *la doctora* was in the know, and for her I wouldn't have to be the arbiter of success and failure. She was informed and wanted to bet on the long shot that she would luck out and live out the months she needed, long enough to see her son graduate. I could see myself fighting for that chance in her situation. That's why she came to California after being turned away from cancer centres on the Eastern Seaboard. Her family had sold what they could just to make the trip from Puerto Rico to Los Angeles to see me. Her retired father was going to sell his home for this. They were putting it all out there to buy a few more moments and some relief from the gnawing, lacerating pain she was experiencing.

Because they were paying out of pocket, I took her to an inexpensive hospital in East LA. I did the operation there so she wouldn't have a bill that would force her family to lose their homes. I also doubled down by bringing another MD / Ph.D. with the same amount of training I had and, more importantly, was an equally capable neurosurgeon. We had pioneered a new dual-surgeon approach for complex cases and extremely ailing patients. Like me, he asked for nothing, out of principle. But it was never about the money. It was about the glory.

I had chosen the day and the team – two anaesthesiologists, two surgeons, two nurses, two runners to grab what we needed and one patient – *la doctora*. I got there before them to set up, and I think it was unlike anything they had seen before. I was moving rubbish bins around, clearing the counters and organizing the cabinets that held the back-up instruments. I was adding specificity to the moment, the moment that might arise when I had to call out for what I needed, and needed fast. Crisis preparation before crisis occurrence. Having those details taken care of allowed me to focus: the preparation is the starting point. No heroics come by accident.

I wanted to leave nothing to chance with *la doctora*. In addition to doubling up on the usual cast and crew, we would perform the surgery with the benefit of a neuromonitoring technician who came in to wire up electrodes all over her body. By then she was 'tubed' with a ventilator hose in her lungs, and 'lined up' with girthy IVs that had been inserted in her neck veins, the internal jugular.

Then we took 'baselines', measurements of electrical connectivity, from the crown of the skull to the tips of the toes. The technician sent electricity into her scalp and brain to see if the leg electrodes detected the signals. If they did, this was proof that the brain and the body were connected electrically, even though the patient was 'asleep'. Then I took off the halo and replaced it with a different crown of metal and puncturing pins that would allow her upper body to be suspended firmly in place over the operating table. *La doctora*'s head and neck were so flimsily bound it was mostly flesh, not skeleton, holding them together.

Next, we needed to rotate her body, very carefully, from being face up to face down, into position, ready for surgery. Given how brittle her neck was, this alone could kill her. Five people were at the ready to twist her body on to her front on the operating table. Two people on the legs, one turning and one catching, same for her torso, and me at the head. Once she was safely in position, an incision was made along the back of her neck from the top of her head to between her shoulder blades. After we'd cut and completed the exposure, we could see the tumour. What we were doing felt more fraught than defusing a bomb. We weren't trying to determine which wires to cut to safely disarm an explosive. We were trying to remove the bomb from the wires without cutting the wires.

That wasn't all. We had to take into consideration the paired vertebral arteries, which arise from the heart and then meander through the bones of the spine and coalesce into the basilary artery – the rare artery that ends almost in a dead end. Disrupting the flow from one of the vertebral arteries into the singular basilar places the reptilian brain at risk of stroke. Patients with brainstem strokes sometimes never wake up and other times wake up but are locked in – conscious but unable to move any muscle but the eyelids, to blink.

I'm not sure why I felt so calm and in my skin. It is a feeling more compelling than a simple surge or rush. Maybe that's what was so addictive. The work was not some ecstatic feeling but something closer to a dissolution of my sense of self. My focus was entirely directed towards the release of movements and the manoeuvres I would perform. The dissection took hours, but it felt like minutes. I was thriving on the pressure. And then, five hours later, we had removed the tumour and *la doctora* was for a moment free of her cancer. She gave me a gift – to learn the deeper meaning that comes from my craft. The most elusive flow state, where mind and body are in synch.

However, there was more to do. The patient's head and neck were wobbly to begin with, and the dissection, though successful, had made it worse. She would require a reconstruction using titanium screws and rods to provide internal seismic retrofitting. The highest two bones of our spine are so uniquely shaped and relevant they are called atlas and axis, as if they belong in mythology. Connecting the patient's skull to this part of her spine would give her head the support it needed. The radiotherapy she had been through before considering surgery had made the course of the artery more tortuous, and when I made the pilot hole for the final screw, I drilled into one of the vertebral arteries. The injury was in such a small orifice in the bone that high-pressure arterial blood squirted out so hard it almost sounded like it was squealing. I quickly rotated my face to the left and the spray hit my ear. I could feel the warm blood dripping down my ear lobe. I put my finger over the hole then rolled my head back and someone in the room gently patted my head with a towel. No communication needed.

The patient's blood pressure dropped, and my team took up their positions. We spent two hours trying to fix the artery, hoping not to have to sacrifice it, but to no avail. The only thing I could do was a bail-out manoeuvre. I placed the long metal screw into the hole and turned it into the bone and into the artery as well, occluding the vessel inside the bone. It was the clinically accepted move in this situation, but it raised the question of whether the remaining blood flow from its partner artery would be enough. We didn't have to wait long.

After ninety seconds the neuromonitoring technician said, 'I'm not getting signals any more from one of the legs.' I said to run them again, after telling the anaesthesiologists to drive up the blood pressure with adrenaline from a syringe. Despite a little extra flow and pressure in the vasculature, there was still no cross coverage, and parts of the brainstem died three minutes later. Some of the brain's signals weren't making it out of the patient's skull. That's why the signals went silent in her leg. I knew *la doctora* would be hurt, but not to what extent. I also knew I'd probably created islands of death in her reptilian brain that covered more than leg function. I was deeply worried that the clusters related to consciousness had been hit. I'd have to wait until she woke up before I knew. No number of electrodes or neuromonitoring on a screen could reveal that kind of information.

Her family, outside, were on edge. I let them know she was alive but that we were waiting a while to see what type and degree of injury she had suffered. It was a long hour.

After *la doctora* woke up, we were able to assess the damage. She had lost all movement in her left leg, and her left arm was weak. I had been preparing myself for the worst-case outcome. I was relieved that she had woken up at all. And I knew we had pulled off something new, not perfectly, but we had made progress. The injury showed how perilous the journey had been.

La doctora was pain free for a while. Even with the halo now off, she needed a wheelchair. Death arrived ten months later, but not before she had taken one last photo with her son at his graduation. For her and her family, hope had been delivered. Her family was deeply appreciative and wrote with updates. The case got me a promotion and a reputation in the circles that mattered to me then, the opinion of surgical masters. Still I wasn't satisfied. I'd stumbled on the last hurdle when I'd had the lead. I could do better. Addiction.

In my interior life, I was chronically unable to steer positive thoughts or accept accolades. I did try. I was a rogue teenager who surprised everyone with a college admission. Then surprised everyone again with a medical school admission after initially struggling in college. But it wasn't until I had a kid and then hurt a kid – Karina – in the space of a year that something raw, something filled with self-hatred, took root and grew. Just getting a college degree after dropping out should be plenty. Sliding into medical school should be plenty. In fact, many med students tend to collapse in terms of ambition because they grab that cocktail-party title – physician – to alleviate some of their social anxiety. But for me, as the competition sharpened, my ambition grew. I could never see what I had already defied, defeated. I only saw those around me, and their bravado, and I wanted to dent their facade. I wanted them to recognize my dominance in an arena where intelligence was necessary but not sufficient. Performance under pressure was the rare ability, the undeniable achievement.

I always had a feeling of being underestimated. I've carried this since my earliest memories. Clearly, there isn't a global conspiracy against me, but every slight, every underestimation, felt like an affront. Most of what I did early on in my life was to prove other people wrong, to make people struggle with their judgements of me. It wasn't as if I felt I was better than everyone else, it wasn't as if I felt like I was more talented than most, it was a feeling of not having reached my potential. Strangely, having an opponent – real or constructed – was a source of energy, a source of drive. A pathological mix of narcissism and insecurity.

It was a flaw in me. It wasn't my upbringing. It wasn't any trauma I had suffered. It was me. Something in my brain, something in my insula maybe, primed me to react in a certain way, and it was getting in the way of the life I wanted to live. My brain was at once the passenger and the driver of my mind. That's the craziest part – that we are both of our brains but above our brains. It makes our minds, but our minds can drift off and return to change our brains. The brain is the only thing that is itself *and* something above it, something free but also partly constrained – like a kite. It is tethered by neurobiology but floats and dances above it. We are thinking flesh. The greatest mystery of the universe.

To appreciate how ambition can be as addictive as a drug, consider the neuroscience of gambling. Gamblers ingest no chemicals, but they experience the same buzz and crash and irrational behaviour as the junkie. Gambling hacks into the brain's pharmacy. True addictions have no endpoint. There is no summit. There is only the next craving and the elusive next high.

My addiction was a bit different. I found a way to take the toxic, destructive elements in my disposition and deliver them for a purpose. Or maybe that's what I prefer to believe. I wanted to be perfect to prove to myself that I wasn't a mediocre surgeon who had injured a child. Then the addiction really took hold, by taking on and working on cases that others couldn't do. Even addictions that don't lead to medical issues can have a tug that disrupts life and relationships, becoming a current that takes too much energy to oppose. The high was something so intense. It was an experience unparalleled, reminding me of what I was capable of, of the potential inside all of us, to anyone willing to use the release of a focused mind.

The brain's reward system, with its reliance on dopamine, has been oversimplified with phrases such as 'dopamine hits'. The system isn't designed so we mindlessly crave rewards, like a rat getting a treat for making it through the maze or someone choosing cocaine over food. It's more of a double-edged sword. Not only can it drive destructive behaviour when left unmanaged by our prefrontal cortex, it can drive long-term coping behaviour as well. The reward system gives us incentives for living well and finding constructive habits attractive, too, just as a damaged reward system can lead to blunted affect and with-drawal from potentially healing behaviour. The hope and anticipation of something positive is its strongest trigger.

After Karina, there was a crater, a primal wound that threw off my neurochemistry and tore down the house of cards I'd constructed out of success and prestige. What happened with Karina became a thorn in my psyche that I carried for over a decade. Trying to find emotional solutions. Trying to find spiritual solutions. This was my private angst, twisting my thoughts. I started wishing for a daughter so I could name her Karina. No shortcuts exist. I started per-forming and teaching paediatric neurosurgery in developing countries as a way to heal this wound, to sever myself from this shame. But even that evolved into something that provided buzz and credit, despite its more heartfelt intentions.

My addiction evaporated with an unforgettable patient. Someone I was deeply close to. A patient who wasn't even under my surgical care. That patient was my father. My father died from medical complications after routine surgery a few years ago. And because of this unexpected death, and because, even if surgery is possible, healing is so much more complicated, I came to see my profession, and my role in it, in a new light. I stopped finding a thrill in doing bigger, more danger-ous surgeries. I no longer sought out the big whack. I now find the term repugnant because it has nothing to do with the patient. Surgeons use it only in the context of how other surgeons perceive the conquest. I started revelling in the craft of surgery, not the glory of it. I didn't need the emotion and intensity attached to it. I came to realize that so much was outside my control, so I should put my best foot forward and enjoy the vicissitudes of life. Be an artisan. Simplify. Embrace the patients and question the system. I realized that surgery is not the mountaintop. The patient's journey is the mountaintop.

Be aware of the rewards you seek in your life and ask yourself what motivates those desires. Are they destructive? Our brains are geared to chase rewards. It's what propels our lives forward. Without drive, our lives lack initiative or direction. We are becalmed on a windless sea. But we also need to manage our desires. We need to be conscious of them, examine them and, ultimately, direct them. Once we lose that internal control, we are addicted.

Addiction was a false passage in my life. My decades-long drive has left me with a rare repertoire of skills, and I now enjoy deploying them on occasion, as patients need them. I like doing basic surgical care as well, which I didn't before. I like doing a difficult case, when I get to operate in my flow, but I've learned I can only do so much. And to appreciate the surgical care of patients, and not use it to indulge my insecurities. I find a deep satisfaction in cutting out cancers when it can help the patient and if they choose it, and

I now take the societal and professional constructs out of the equation. I'm learning to core down to the essential. Patient and surgeon. What we share is life-affirming, especially when the stakes are high.

8.

Stress

Would you give a blood transfusion to keep a girl from dying? What if the girl's parents believed a transfusion would be going against the will of their god and deliver her to eternal pain?

The first time I saw Elena and her parents, I didn't think I'd face this choice. She was diagnosed with a hemangioblastoma, one of several children's brain cancers and the least aggressive of the group. Surgery can completely cure a hemangioblastoma by removing the tumour. Sometimes, in cases like this, cancer surgeons have a rare opportunity to take out a tumour entirely and leave the patient perfect.

With Elena's surgery, I'd need to shell all of the tumour out and leave no trace behind. At the same time, I'd need to avoid injuring neuronal tissue. It's hard to get both done, but that is why cases like these present the perfect challenge: a surgeon's technical skill alone determines the outcome. The four possible outcomes were: cured but injured, not cured but perfect, not cured and injured, or cured and perfect. Do it right, and the surgery wouldn't require any subsequent treatments, no collaboration with physicians offering chemotherapy and radiation.

When we met, Elena's parents informed me that they were Jehovah's Witnesses and would not allow their daughter to receive a blood transfusion. They were clear: no blood, under no circumstance. I respected their faith and I had no intention of disrespecting any loving parents' wishes. For Jehovah's Witnesses, the prohibition against blood transfusions comes from biblical passages that forbid eating blood. They consider a transfusion to be another form of eating and liken a blood transfusion to someone being fed through a feeding tube. Going against this prohibition is no small matter for Jehovah's Witnesses. In fact, the stakes could not be higher. According to the religion's website: 'It is out of obedience to the highest authority in the universe, the Creator of life . . . Their relationship with their Creator and God is at stake.'

The weird thing was that Elena's parents weren't at all what I expected, with the prejudices I'd absorbed. They looked no different from other affluent people in Los Angeles. They said they were Jehovah's Witnesses and that they'd come to me because they'd heard from an elder in their church that I could get the work done with the least blood loss. Fast surgeons lose less blood because we know what we're doing and can complete the work with fewer steps. Elena's parents brought so much paperwork with them for me to review, I thought I was buying a house.

The London Regional Transfusion Committee has an extensive flow chart and multiple checklists for managing patients who don't want blood transfusions. The chart affects things big – estimating blood loss ahead of time – and small: recommending the use of paediatric tubes for adult blood samples. There is also a list of blood products that the patient has to go through, marking which they accept and which they reject. The checklist includes red blood cells, platelets, fresh frozen plasma, cryoprecipitate, albumin, recombinant clotting factors and fibrinogen concentrate. These are the individual components of whole blood.

There are a few modifications to the strict prohibition of blood transfusions for those of the Jehovah's Witness faith. If the patient's total blood cells run low, the blood pressure can be maintained by transfusing saline to keep the vessels from quivering and collapsing. This doesn't help deliver oxygen to tissue, but it does mean the vessels remain patent, allowing the existing red blood cells to deliver what they can. Jehovah's Witnesses are usually OK with this. Some will ask for permission within the church to allow for erythropoietin. EPO, as it is known, stimulates red blood cell production in the bone marrow. Cancer patients undergoing chemotherapy take EPO to boost their plunging red blood cell levels. Athletes have also taken it to give themselves an illegal edge on the competition, a pharmacological substitute for training at high altitude.

Elena had Von Hippel-Lindau Syndrome, a rare genetic condition that prompts the body to make extra EPO. In her case, the syndrome had also resulted in tumours sprouting in wide expanses of her body. She'd inherited the condition from her father. As a result of her Von Hippel-Lindau Syndrome, she had a tumour in the back of her brain and one on top of her kidney, in the adrenal gland. The brain tumour had a bright perimeter with a dark interior and a little bright white nodule tucked away like an alien embryo in amniotic fluid. This tumour is even able to create its own fertilizer, manipulating cellular DNA to crank out both VEGF, a vascular growth factor, which makes blood vessels sprout, and EPO, the protein that tells your bone marrow to create and release more red blood cells. This meant two things: the tumour was going to have a lot of extra vessels feeding it, and it was leaking EPO into the global arterial system. As a result, Elena had a high hematocrit, the ratio of red blood cells to total blood volume, which provided a built-in advantage. The greater number of red blood cells meant she'd be able to supply her organs with enough oxygen even if she lost some blood.

There are over a hundred forms of brain surgery, and it can be hit and miss whether or not the patient is going to need a blood transfusion. Some cases, we know going in that they can get bloody, so we have a stock of the patient's blood type at the ready. Others catch us by surprise, and we give them universal donor blood, O negative, as this blood won't trigger anyone's immune response. Either way, we don't lose people because there isn't enough blood. Death on the operating table happens because the blood isn't going in as fast as it is coming out. We also know that children can't handle blood loss as well as adults.

In Elena's case, her brain tumour had a sibling nestled in the adrenal glands. The adrenal glands release cortisol, known in simple terms as the stress hormone. The brain commands a variety of glands by slipping hormones out of the pituitary, the master hormone regulator, which sits straight back from the bridge of your nose. The pituitary, in turn, listens to the hypothalamus, which sits above it. The three-step hypothalamus-pituitary-adrenal (HPA) axis provides several dials to fine-tune the mixture of neurochemicals and hormones that constantly circulate inside us. But those dials are not autonomous from your thoughts and intentions. The prefrontal cortex sits above it all and has evolved descending neuronal branches to adjust those knobs that modulate the HPA and thereby our ultimate response to stressors.

Hijacked by a tumour, Elena's adrenal glands were firing autonomously, without the usual signals from the pituitary. She was hitting on all cylinders, a stress response without stress. Even though her body acted as though it was under stress, Elena didn't feel stressed. Her prefrontal cortex took care of that. Her thinking brain determined that there was no cause for stress and psychologically ignored her body's surging adrenaline and sky-high blood pressure.

Before surgery, though, we needed to turn down this rush of adrenaline. Otherwise, the stress of surgery could result in blood pressure so high multiple arteries throughout the body would pop, a condition called malignant hypertension. We did this by giving Elena propranolol, a medication that blocks the receptors on the blood vessels and heart, turning down some of the dials on her runaway stress response. Propranolol lowers blood pressure and has also been used to help people forget their trauma.

During the surgery Elena was in a sitting position, the operating table configured into a chair, as metal pins kept her torso propped up and her head upright even though she was unconscious. Gravity would be an advantage, revealing corridors unavailable when the patient is horizontal. During the exposure, I hadn't even got to the tumour before an underappreciated enemy struck. The back of the brain has thinner dura concealing the veins. The usual quick drilling you'd use on other parts of the skull isn't possible, so I began the surgery by eggshelling Elena's skull. With a fine drill with diamond-tipped burrs I painted away the bone of her skull until her skull was eggshell thin, hence the name. Then, with fine, chisel-like instruments, the last vestige of the skull was delicately lifted. Despite the cautious approach, when

I did this I tore off a bit of her torcular Herophili, the spot where three major veins come to a confluence and then descend through the left and right jugular veins, draining blood from the brain to the heart.

I could fix this. It would be challenging, but it was far from impossible. But, doing it without the luxury of being able to replace blood added to the challenge. I needed to place forty to fifty fine stitches, sewing the edges of the tear together, starting from the intact edges, the untorn edges, then zip both sides inwards to a final double stitch in the middle. Because the veins are broad and floppy, I had to make sure my stitches didn't go through both sides of the vessel. I also needed to work fast. In between each stitch the vessel would have to be allowed to flow to irrigate Elena's brain. It's like working underwater on a leaking pipe; blood is flowing, making it hard to get the next stitch in. Then you have to repeat the steps again and again and again. Through each manoeuvre, she would drop more blood, but because of her tumour she came tanked up with extra blood. Totally manageable, I was telling myself. I was trying to reassure myself, but I could feel my emotions closing in. To do my best work, I needed to regulate my emotions as I placed the stitches.

For me, the key step to controlling my emotions is recognizing that my attention can be turned inwards, to think about the emotions I am feeling. We need to be conscious of our emotions in order to be able to guide them. We want our emotions to match the situation. It's a common misimpression that surgeons have to learn to disconnect themselves from their emotions to be able to do what we do. In fact, the opposite is true for me. The emotional weight of knowing the person under the surgical drape elevates my performance, brings me fully to the moment.

I went through thirty minutes of stitch work, tying a knot after each throw of the needle with one hand, four knots on each thread so there was no chance of the stitches unravelling. I was quick and thorough, but with each manoeuvre I was running out of fuel, and the runway remained distant. Elena's life wouldn't be at stake if we had been able to give her some blood to make up for what she was losing as we stitched. In that case, there would be no risk of death in the operating theatre, but what it took to get this stitch work done mattered deeply to her parents. From their perspective, nothing less than her soul was on the line. The pressure was building steadily, and the weight of it was now pressing down on me.

We need stress in life. If we don't have enough stress, we become brittle. Too much, and we break. This is true at the cellular level, too. Not enough stress, and stem cells in the brain won't gestate and release new brain cells. Too much stress, and they prefer dormancy. The emotional and cognitive brains are not independent but are literally connected by overlapping neuronal branching. Emotion and cognition are designed to be reciprocal. They co-evolved, and we are at our best when there is a dynamic equilibrium between reason and emotion.

Understanding these intertwining forests in the brain, old and new, emotion and cognition, offers a lifelong opportunity for self-regulation. Squash all emotion, and we lose our instinct. We can no longer react quickly and feel deeply. Let emotion run amok, and we're unable to focus and reason. For most of us, improving self-regulation means the cognitive brain reining in our emotional selves. Our ancient, emotional brain leans a little loose and wild. It's not biased towards focusing on the negative. It is biased towards vigilance, even hypervigilance. It's uncertainty and pattern disruption that perk up our antennae, and these are neither negative nor positive. That's why it's hard to acclimatize to sporadic threats. Calibrating this vigilance is an essential feature of stress management and emotional regulation.

Stressors can disrupt and even sever these emotional–cognitive connections, leading to unchecked emotions. As a result, emotional regulation takes more and more effort. This downward spiral can lead to perpetual stress and anxiety, sapping our ability to focus and wasting our cognitive reserve.

Elena's red blood cell count at the start was above normal, thanks to the EPO her tumour was releasing into her system. The confluence of three giant veins in the brain at the torcula sheds blood fast, but not faster than we can replace it. The brain is the only part of the body where veins can't be simply singed shut or clamped off. Surgeons routinely disrespect veins in the rest of the body because there are so many alternative routes returning used blood to the heart. The brain is different. Almost every vessel is critical in the brain.

Elena's blood pressure was sinking, even though I'd told the anaesthesiologist to stop the drug that was holding back the adrenaline. Her heart rate was not going up. The measurements showed that she was 'dry', which meant her fluids had not been topped up enough. But she needed more than just saline, she needed blood.

The inevitable question was now upon us: do we go against her family's wishes to save her life? Technically, Elena wasn't going to bleed to death, but the heart needs a certain engorgement to function. After enough blood loss, the heart begins to quiver into a deadly arrhythmia. Without a blood transfusion soon, the patient would die. If she had been an adult and had insisted on not receiving a blood transfusion, I would have let her go. I did not feel the same way about a child. However, her parents had the legal right to make that call, and Elena would die if I followed their wishes. I said we needed to seriously consider giving her blood, and now.

The senior nurse said she didn't want to be a part of it. The anaesthesiologist was also against it. He said, 'We need to respect the parents' wishes.' To me, that was nuts. Elena was in trouble, and the room had unexpectedly sided with the parents. They'd only met her and her parents that morning, for a few minutes. They hadn't been there for the multiple clinic visits. They wouldn't be there for the aftermath.

At the time, I was still struggling with what had happened with Karina, so this felt like opening up a psychological wound that hadn't yet finished festering. Those emotions and memories coloured my thinking about what to do. Maybe I was partly trying to fix a past mistake. With Karina, I went for a textbook solution rather than listening to my instincts. In the end, responding under pressure rarely delivers a hero's tale. Sometimes, it just means remaining true to who you believe yourself to be. I was going to go with my gut. Giving Elena blood was the only solution that felt true to me, to who I am. In this case, though, I put myself above her parents. I'm not sure if I would have given her blood if the shame and regret I felt after Karina's case hadn't been colouring my thoughts. It's hard to say. Maybe, in that moment, saving myself was also important. Elena would live, but my response would be self-serving.

Pressure is there because the outcome matters to us and, in this case, I would be punished either way. Give Elena blood and go against her parents' unwavering religious directive. Don't give her blood and lose her on the operating table. Strangely, saving her life

would probably hurt my career. Like my confrontation with the professor, protecting my *self* might
mean risking my livelihood. For Elena's parents,
saving their child almost meant losing their child, and
they would probably grieve at the thought of their
daughter losing her afterlife.

While my partner watched the surgical field, I
went out into the hallway and grabbed two units of
O negative blood. Come on, you can't be banished
from heaven for two units of blood, I tried to tell
myself. I connected it to her IV and squeezed it
myself. I squeezed it like this was a trauma case. No
one could say the staff were pressured. The pressure
was all mine as I squeezed that blood bag. Maybe it
was selfish, but I couldn't handle what letting a girl
die because of my mistake would do to my self-
narrative. A few hours later, with the vessel repaired,
the surgery was over and Elena's tumour was out.

When I approached her parents after completing
the surgery, I could feel the tension on their faces. I
said, 'I did run into some complications, but Elena is
fine, awake, talking and moving.' When I finished
this first sentence their expression went from being
braced for bad news to relief. The muscles around
their eyes relaxed, their chests deflated, releasing the
nervous inhalation, all the pressure in them subsided.
I hadn't finished, though.

I said, 'I did have to give two units of blood,' adding,
'O negative, the universal donor,' as if this would

make the blood less dirty in their minds, as if it would mean that I hadn't sullied their daughter in the eyes of their Creator. Elena's parents' expressions went from relief to affront, filled with indignation at my crime. They were mortified.

A fate worse than death is how they saw it. I thought they would still be relieved that their daughter's life had been saved, in spite of their clearly explained and documented wishes. Faced with the choice of their girl dying on the operating table on my watch and violating their religion, I had made the only choice I could live with. Our surgical consent paperwork allows for 'intraoperative' decisions. Frankly, surgeons have been using the 'intraoperative decisions' clause as a dodge when they make a mistake – sometimes injuring patients by their own hand and sometimes by not getting the planned work done, something we derisively call 'peek and shriek'. But that wasn't what happened with this case. I fixed the surgical complication and removed the tumour but left Elena's family in a spiritual crisis. I put myself first, and I think her parents knew that.

As a result of my decision, the hospital sought a lawyer, a case manager and a patient advocate to look into the surgery. The family threatened to report me to the medical board. It was a strange public shaming but, in that crucible of incredible stress, I knew I couldn't have lived with the death of this girl. But there was a lasting consequence: this was the last case

I ever did involving a Jehovah's Witness. The community no longer referred patients to me. News of my transgression spread.

There are stressful situations we find ourselves in, as I did with the Jehovah's Witness family. But there are also stressful relationships that are imposed on us by others. After I had blocked the professor in the operating theatre years earlier, he put me on probation for 'endangering a patient's life' and had me on the precipice of termination. The following Tuesday, he was back in the operating theatre. Tuesday was a sought-after day to schedule surgeries because the patient was usually discharged before the weekend, thereby relieving the surgeon of having to come in on a Saturday or Sunday to see them. The professor was allowed to pick anyone he wanted to join him in the operating theatre. In many jobs, getting face time with the boss would be deemed a bonus. Not so with the professor because he could – and did – fire anyone he didn't like. Working with him was not viewed as a plum assignment, an opportunity to learn from the head honcho, but as a liability, a chance to wind up in his crosshairs. I only had a spot in neurosurgery in the first place because the professor had fired a trainee, creating a vacancy. He fired two other trainees during my seven years under him.

That Tuesday after Karina's surgery, the professor requested that I join him in the operating theatre at his next surgery. And so it began. From that point on, he kept asking me to be assigned to his cases. He kept booking more complicated cases. Operations he couldn't do on his own and which should have been assigned to other, more competent professors. Operations I had never done before. And when I raised concerns about the danger of this arrangement for the patients, I was repeatedly fired then rehired weeks later, to keep me in line.

I became hypervigilant, in threat mode, marinating in HPA toxicity under his mercurial ways. It was exhilarating and disconcerting. At the weekends, I would go and practise on the anatomy cadavers used for training medical students. I remember drilling out the optic canal and optic strut on a cadaver one Saturday, getting ready for a surgery a couple of days away. I'd stayed away from the cadavers during medical school. I'd hated the smell of formaldehyde, and the first-year students were like vultures huddled over bodies. Those cadavers I never once touched as a medical student were now my GPS, a chance to practise some of the things I'd need to do on the living in a couple of days.

With the professor, my role in the cases I did with him was kept from the patients and their families. The professor would meet with them before and after surgery and pretend he was handling the case solo. I would lurk on the fire stairs that led to the operating theatre. I'd go in and do the surgery then vanish. The operating theatre nurses started calling me Ghost. Taking the helm in complicated cases makes you a better surgeon – or it reveals an irreparable flaw: that one can't perform under pressure. I blossomed under pressure, and I benefited from the experience, but it wasn't fair to the unwitting patients.

The practice of allowing trainees to operate at the edge of their skill level or beyond persists. And it happens far more often than you might want to think. Since we weren't creating obvious injuries and showing up in M&Ms, no one stepped in to make the professor stop. It became an open secret in our department, hidden from his superiors at the university. Sadly, the year after I graduated, when the professor was operating alone, he injured so many patients that the university took away his privileges to operate. In my absence, he kept signing up patients for surgery who thought they were getting a prestigious surgeon, but he no longer had the surreptitious back-up to save him from his mistakes. The stress of this relationship and experience was extreme and had put me under immense pressure, but it also taught me a great deal.

To manage the pressure of working like this with the surgeon for three years, I started running the list, just as we 'ran the list' of the sickest patients in the morning. Before heading into the operating theatre, I would run the list on my priorities: my sons' health, providing for my family, and so on. This cognitive distancing helped to stop me from catastrophizing. This worked to relieve some of the pressure, to ease some of the worry and anxiety as I headed in to perform surgery in which I was going to have to perform past my ability and in secret. Under pressure, the true skill is not to heighten focus, but to reduce distraction.

Possibility and uncertainty walk hand in hand, so a bit of anxiety is an essential element of a successful life. Certainly, my baptism of fire with the professor showed me my potential surgical abilities. Challenging or difficult circumstances provoke a physiological response. In the short term, this helps us rise to the occasion. If we face chronic stress, however, this same response will injure both body and brain. For years, I was always in over my depth. I learned to fly blind. I did it, and I feel survivor's guilt for it still. Being pulled into the deep end before I was ready was the rarest of life lessons.

Stress has to occur, precisely because, without it, there can be no growth. The management of stress is an ability rooted in neurobiology within us, but it must be cultivated consciously. Whenever one is in a stressful situation, the essential step is to take time to turn your attention inwards. Expand the vocabulary by which you describe your feelings to yourself. Let your emotions earn a place in your mind. Contest and dispute your emotions if needed, but release them, too. We must regulate our emotions regularly or stress will spiral in a direction where it becomes a constant, requiring no trigger or activation. A baseline of unwell being.

Remarkably, your efforts to balance thought and emotion in times of stress lead to the birth of new neurons to help you in this cause. These new neurons are allies and help you regulate your emotions and re-establish calm. And it explains why successfully managing stress makes it easier to manage stress in the future, allowing us to cope and thrive where, once, we may have struggled.

9.

Loss

By 2003, I had a mere twelve months of training under my belt. I was a medical doctor with an MD after my name. I felt that medical technicians and pool lifeguards knew more than I did, but now I was wearing that long white coat, everyone but the senior surgeons had to listen. I wasn't giving many orders, though. The first year of surgical training doesn't offer any surgical experience. We rarely went into the operating theatre. I thought this made the first year of training a waste.

I did learn something about my limitations: I was developing an instinct as to when I should handle issues on my own and when I should bump it up the chain of command. Hospitals are all about the chain of command. Nurses call trainees. Trainees call professors, and professors call other specialists when patients develop issues outside their expertise. The first year isn't about being a doctor, it's about mastering multitasking.

I was also beginning to learn about hospital turf wars. Most parts of the body have two types of experts, one surgical and one medical. Cardiac surgeons are complemented by cardiologists, liver surgeons by hepatologists, kidney surgeons by nephrologists, lung surgeons by pulmonologists. Often these doctors work together. Just as often, they butt heads. The hospital is filled with bickering services. Doctors and surgeons argue about what the next step of management should be for patients with complicated cases, often taking any professional disagreement personally. Typically, the team with the most historical clout have their way in patient care when multiple services and opinions are involved. As I was doing my best to learn the nuances of these various warring tribes, one surgeon seemed above the fray, a transplant surgeon named Greg.

'If there's an organ donor, want to go?' he asked one day. I didn't need to answer. He knew me by then.

Two weeks later, Greg called and asked me to go to the hospital and get one of our patients waiting for a liver set up with lines that would give access into major veins. Her lucky day had arrived. A donor had been found. Patients have to be readied for transplant surgery ahead of time. Sometimes, patients are prepped for surgery and the donated organs turn out to be unsuitable, so they have to go back to the hospital floor and resume their lives. The ones in hospital were the sickest patients, there for months and months, awaiting a transplant. Other, less sick, liver patients stay at home, waiting to get a call that their time is now.

Once the patient was ready, Greg came up to the fifth floor and said, 'Let's go.' The organs were in Santa Fe, New Mexico, so we needed to get airborne fast. Downstairs, a driver in a black sedan with tinted windows was waiting. We got in the back seat. When we arrived at the airport, we skipped the terminal. The driver pulled straight on to the tarmac, where a Learjet was waiting. It all seemed very gangster, but there was a good reason for the rushed getaway. Organs have a very short shelf life. They rot with time. So, we couldn't fly commercial with the organs once we'd harvested them, nor could we take a prop plane for the almost 750-mile flight back.

We arrived in Santa Fe and walked into a little community hospital. Security escorted us up in the lift to the ICU. I pushed the large button on the wall with my knuckles to keep my fingertips clean and the familiar double doors opened. The scene that awaited me was anything but familiar, to me anyway. The nurses eyed us as we entered. We were strangers in their hospital, foreigners in their domain, and they knew why we were there. No doubt a nurse among them had done what she could for weeks to fend off this young man's death, cared for him in the way she would want her younger brother treated. Maybe she had cried with the family. Our job was different. The only finesse and care we brought would be in the form of surgical technique.

Greg and I found the man lying alone in an ICU

room. He was nineteen, technically an adult, but he seemed much too young for what was about to happen. In the US, he was not old enough legally to drink alcohol, but he was about to be disassembled. His family had gone. They had said their last goodbyes. He was still on a ventilator, brain dead, but his body was alive – kept alive for us. I wasn't that much older than he was, at twenty-seven. The young man's heart was pumping like those of the other ICU patients but, unlike them, his heart was not supplying blood to his brain. Those blood vessels were clotted off, cemented with scabs on the inside: no cerebral blood flow, the undeniable stigmata of brain death. There was a macabre energy to the room. We were like the zombie squad, walking into someone else's home to steal a loved one, to bring an end to his short life.

Psychiatrist Elisabeth Kübler-Ross was a pioneer in the study of death and dying. She described the five progressive stages of grief: denial, anger, bargaining, depression and acceptance. This young man's family were grieving. I wondered where on the Kübler-Ross continuum they were. Were they still feeling the frustration, irritation and anxiety related to anger? Or had they moved on to bargaining and a struggle to find acceptance? Or were they still being thrashed around by all those 'stages' at once, in an unnavigable mix of pain and suffering? In her final book, Kübler-Ross took a more nuanced view: 'Our loss is as individual as our lives.'

After a public tragedy, there's always talk in the media of bringing closure to the grieving, as if a loved one's life is a book that can be placed on a shelf. Parents who have lost a child will tell you there's no such thing as closure. Beyond the most fundamental biological bonds, a lifetime's web of memories connects parent and child. Death doesn't sever these, nor should we ask parents – or any loved one – to seek closure on the death of a loved one. Life moves on, but the connections remain, indelible memories that have a physical presence in the brain. The grieving shouldn't be asked to forget their grief, nor can they, but they need to remember that the loss of a loved one is a trauma. Like other traumas, it must be confronted and framed in a way that makes it possible to function in the world.

For advanced cancer patients, their diagnosis forces a different reckoning: the loss of the life they imagined having. Instead of a life that ends in old age, they face a new life that is shorter, syncopated with hospital stays and uncertainty, with treatments and pain. Surprisingly, many do not end up viewing cancer as a loss at all. For them, the unexpected final chapter is not a requiem, a coda to their pre-cancerous life, but a fuller existence in spite of their illness; they are focused on what matters.

When threatened with a cataclysm, Proust writes, we immediately see where our priorities should be. Once the threat passes, 'We find ourselves back in the heart of normal life, where negligence deadens desire. And yet we shouldn't have needed the cataclysm to love life today. It would have been enough to think that we are humans and that death might come this evening.' For cancer patients, they are living inside the cataclysm. Cancer patients have shown me that having 'quality of life' is not just a priority but *the* priority.

As we pushed the gurney out of the ICU room and into the hallway, I had no idea what had mattered to the young man, how he had lived his life, or what he or his family had planned for his now lost future. The nurses caring for patients in the other rooms paused and came closer to the wide doors that fed out of each individual room. Some were crying. I didn't know what emotion provoked the tears. Relief? Revulsion? Some indecipherable mixture of the two? As we passed, the nurses gave us sidelong glances, as if we were accomplices in this young man's death, and, in a way, we were. They avoided eye contact, and I couldn't help thinking that they somehow looked simultaneously grateful that we were there and disgusted by us. I'd never been looked at like that before, and I haven't since.

We wheeled this warm body through unfamiliar hallways into the operating theatre as if we were trying to save him. Still on the ventilator, the brain-dead young man was then moved to the operating table. The back table was set up with sterile equipment just like in every other operation, but this was anything but. The vibe was different. The cast and crew were quiet. We were there to deliver death on our terms. His death would mean a new life for others. On paper, I was at peace with the maths.

Greg asked me to prep from the man's neck down to his thighs. Usually, patients are prepped with orange disinfecting fluid only in the space where surgeons are planning on cutting, plus a generous margin. In this case, the young man's body was orange from below his jaw to his mid-thigh.

'I'll meet you in the middle,' Greg said. He and I stood on opposite sides of the body. He was going to cut from the patient's groin to where the ribcage parted; I was to cut down from the notch in the middle of the collarbones called the suprasternal.

My experience in the operating theatre at this point was minimal. I felt that I didn't know what I was doing. Greg had to call my instruments for me. After the initial incision, he called for a saw to cut the sternum. The nurse handed me a heavy, grey metal saw with a foot plate like a giant sewing machine and a trigger like one on a power tool. Greg told me to cut in the neck first and then hook the foot plate underneath the sternum and lift the whole way through as though I were trying to pull the young man off the bed. My heart was beating twice as fast as the heart I was about to un-encase. I did it as Greg asked. I had never seen an open chest before.

Underneath a beige, slightly translucent satchel

called the pericardium, the heart looked like a caged monster, a dancer in a straitjacket, explosive and rhythmic. I could see it writhing, not beating but erupting, ejecting, like wringing out a towel. The heart is striking in its ferocity of movement. I could see why for millennia it was considered the seat of our souls.

I tried to shake my admiration and awe and get to the work at hand. For a moment, I was in a trance state. To expose the heart, I had to grab its cape, the thick membrane around it, the pericardium. When the heart squeezes itself, like a fist, it pulls away momentarily from the pericardium and there is just a hint of slack in its skin. That's when I needed to grab the pericardium. I felt for a moment like a conductor, but I quickly realized I wasn't in control. The heart was. I was trying to follow the heart's conduction. I was being hypnotized. With my right hand, I picked up a scalpel. I started thinking about this young man's family, what they had expected from the final minutes of existence for their son, brother, grandson.

My hands were facing down over his spread chest, an instrument dangling softly from each. My movements were in synch with my surroundings. And then I went for it. I plucked the pericardium lightly with the forceps in my left hand and then sliced a little opening with the scalpel in my right. I handed away the narrow scalpel and then slid my right middle finger inside. With my gloved fingernail to the heart's muscular back, I used the pad of a finger to lift the pericardium off the heart. I could see my finger inside the sheath. I let my left hand go and picked up a bovie, an electric knife. I discharged its current, and the sheath around the heart spread. Now I could see its full form. It was like a muscular back that has torn through a well-stitched jacket, like a swimmer's beautiful rippling shoulders.

But I wasn't here to harvest his heart. If this heart had been precious, it wouldn't have been left in my dedicated but immature hands. The young man lying on the table had a heart condition. This vital organ was damaged and could not be transplanted. I was here to lance a chamber in his heart, but only when Greg needed me to. It had to happen at the same time as the harvesting. The organs needed blood until the last possible moment. Then, Greg gave me the nod and I did it. I took a curved pair of scissors and closed the blades around the heart. I felt the muscle dividing as the scissors closed. The texture, the movement, that moment, together are unforgettable.

For minutes, the heart continued to beat. Normally, blood flowing out of the heart meets resistance. That's why there is measurable blood pressure. This young man's heart was now squeezing blood out through a torn wall into open air, the blood flowing like water from an open dam into the ribcage. Greg told me to drop the suction into the chest and come to help him. I moved down from the chest to the belly, but I couldn't stop watching the heart's death throes in my peripheral vision. The young man's brain was dead, but the heart was under the command of nerves that fire autonomously when the brain can't be relied upon.

Despite draining its lifeblood, the heart still squeezed. With its empty, slightly sunken chambers, it looked like a flattened soufflé. The heart no longer followed a rhythmic, predictable beat. Minutes had passed. As the blood flow slowed to a trickle, Greg was busy harvesting the organs.

Even though the heart still fluttered, I had to start closing the chest. I used a surgical plier to stitch with a thick, curved needle trailing a pliable wire. It felt like closing a casket on a breathing person, but I couldn't wait for the heart to be still. The young man's organs were now on ice and the Learjet awaited. I saved time closing the breastbone by being as quick and precise as I could, but I made sure to leave tidy skin stitches in case his family wanted an open casket.

The young man's 'time of death' had officially been recorded minutes earlier, when I lanced his heart, but behind the now-closed breastbone, the heart still had a few shivers left, unseen and unappreciated. So what was his true time of death? Should it have been when the heart was lanced, or when it finally stopped? Or should time of death have been when he lost consciousness for the last time? Or when his family made their final visit? Life has gradations and, as such, death is not given the nuance it deserves.

With our red-and-white Igloo cooler filled with ice and organs, each in their own sealed sterile bag, we boarded the chartered jet to head back home. I sat in the backward-facing seat, the cooler tucked under me. Throughout the flight, I could feel the Igloo becoming colder, the plastic chilling my calves. The organs were now living a brief life of their own, whole but with no master, waiting to find soil or themselves perish. Greg was asleep. A veteran of many trips like this, he was resting in advance of the transplant surgeries ahead and the people who would spring back to life with a transplanted organ. I was awake, trying to understand what had happened.

Back at the hospital in San Diego, we transplanted two kidneys, a pancreas and a liver over the next thirty-six hours. And over those two days operating on four people back to back, I felt exhausted but relieved. All the patients had their new organs grafted successfully.

A few months later I was recruited by Neurosurgery, and Greg never held my decision to leave Transplant against me. I thought I'd left it behind for good but, within months, inspired by my experience in Santa Fe, I would be engaging with it again in a different way.

When I started out in neurosurgery, I was responsible for all non-surgical work. That meant taking care of head trauma patients on machines, brains that didn't need brain surgery ever or just yet, post-surgery patients recovering, and patients on the brink of brain death in the neuro ICU. Also, I was just twenty-seven and mostly pretending to be a neurosurgeon.

While more senior trainees were learning to operate, I was spending my time in the ICU. The intensive care unit is the most challenging medical care, but that's where the most junior neurosurgery trainees are sent, to learn from the most extreme cases. We are expected to hit the ground running. It gives us a lot of confidence to be trusted with such sick patients. These are the same cases seen by advanced trainees in medicine, yet we are the novices in neurosurgery. That's when I learned that all surgeons are physicians, but not all physicians are surgeons.

There are only two hospital teams that can't talk to a patient's families at the same time: Neurosurgery and Organ Transplant. Neurosurgeons declare patients brain dead; transplant surgeons harvest their organs. Talk about conflicting interests. One tries to help patients live, even when the flame is barely flickering. The other sees the benefit in allowing the patient to die. The rationale for requiring transplant surgeons to wait to talk to the donor's family is that, otherwise, they might be a bit hasty to let a patient go since that lets them save up to seven of the lives that are in their mental queue, should all the organs become available. Neurosurgeons who declare 'brain death' aren't supposed to broach organ transplantation, and transplant doctors can't approach the family of a patient until they've elected to discuss organ donation themselves.

I came to understand why this policy was in place –
after I broke it.

Just a few weeks into switching to neurosurgery, I got
the call to the Emergency Department. When I arrived,
the patient's single mother and fiancée were by his side.
He was in his late teens and went by the name of
Edward. The deep basal ganglia in his left hemisphere
had a massive haemorrhage. I had no idea what had
caused it or what would come next. I knew I had to do
a few things quickly. I put him on a breathing machine,
then inserted a catheter to drain fluid and keep the pressure from building up dangerously in his brain.

Imaging showed he had an AVM (arteriovenous
malformation), a strange, tangled ball of blood vessels, arteries and veins, like snakes in a bag, that were
thinner than they should be. AVMs are rare, the cause
unknown, and they can pop up randomly. Edward
had a ruptured AVM. The flow through them was
torrential and turbulent. His mother and fiancée were
caught in the shockwaves. I wasn't much older than
Edward, and I was a new father. His sudden turn for
the worse affected me more than I wanted to admit.

His care during those long weeks in the ICU
ground down hope. I was in the ICU a lot. His mother
was there almost around the clock. Her outward
kindness and strength veiled her grief. His fiancée
was there, too. As a resident, I was pulled in many
directions, but I did pay more attention to Edward
than to other patients.

Three weeks went by, and Edward never woke up. To family members, it seemed as if his condition was unchanged. He was simply 'sleeping on the breathing machine'. The truth was much worse. Parts of his brain had started to die. Parts which manage the nerves that exit the face. Some go to the eyeballs from the optic apparatus deep inside the brain, not only moving them but controlling the pupil. The reptilian brain, the brain-stem, also sends out nerves to the throat, controlling the cough and gag reflexes. What happens with these face nerve functions reveals what is happening in the brain.

Edward's pupils were wide open, dilated in their most relaxed position. When I shone a torch in them, they didn't reflexively close, as they should, to limit the exposure to the bright light. Unresponsive pupils are called fixed. Edward was 'fixed and dilated'. Ominous. When I rocked his head gently left and right, his eyeballs didn't swivel to keep looking straight up, as they should. This reflex is called 'doll's eyes'. Edward's eyes were locked to their sockets. He'd lost his 'doll's eyes', indicating that there were more islands of dead brain. Other tests revealed the devastating damage AVM had done to swathes of Edward's brain.

Even as his brain withered, his most basic instincts persisted. When I stuck a long Q-tip in his throat, Edward gagged. I asked the nurse to suction his lungs through the breathing tube, and he coughed. His mother thought that these were good signs, but I knew her son was trapped in purgatory. He still had a cough and gag reflex, but he was fixed and dilated. Semi-dead, with no chance of recovery. The thinking and emotional parts of his brain were dead. But his brainstem was alive.

The catheter I'd placed through his skull into his brain was the reptilian brain's friend, but this mother's enemy. I wanted to break Edward's fall, but no meaningful action was left. My intervention, the catheter, kept him from a grave that would offer him, his mother and his fiancée some solace.

I knew Edward couldn't hear or understand, or even feel for that matter, but I would say, 'Hi, Edward, this is Dr Jandial, I'm going to check a few things on your face.' Then I would gently poke and prod to check for a cough or a gag.

Where tissue damage occurs in the brain determines whether a patient can bounce back. Damage in some areas is insurmountable. There are no miracles with certain brain injuries. Edward had that kind of injury, and I was watching his gradual demise. His mother didn't know what the tests I was doing meant. To her, they were no different than the nurses checking her son's blood pressure or feeding tube. At best, Edward would live in a 'vegetative state'. What vulgar terminology we trained with, a way to dehumanize the devastated. The term suggested that his life would be less than that of an animal – a vegetable; a squash or a carrot – implying that he was not even sentient. The only thing keeping Edward alive was a catheter in his brain. It had been put there originally to give him a chance, until his fate was declared. Now, Edward's dismal future was clear.

Remembering my experience with transplants, I started to feel that this family's grief could be tempered by only two things: meaning and purpose. Meaning to the meaningless tragedy; purpose to a life cut short. These would help his mother and fiancée find sanity amid the questions that were certain to arise in the years and decades ahead after such a random and tragic turn in their lives. Edward's death could give life to others. His mother knew nothing about organ donation, and I was prohibited from influencing her. He wasn't brain dead, so transplant surgeons weren't allowed to talk to her about what his organs could do for others. I knew about that. I also knew that his brain was profoundly injured and could never meaningfully recover.

I brought his mother down softly and fairly. I delivered the news methodically and authentically. True in good news, and true in bad news. That was how we connected. Death had been delayed temporarily by my catheter and by the machine that pushed breaths into him.

Remember, the hospital forbids transplant surgeons and brain surgeons to talk to each other in such cases. They are linked, but their paths to saving lives are distinct, so there is no collaborating. To understand the options, I met with the hospital ethics committees, which are populated by administrative types who rarely feel the pain of the trenches. And I learned that families can't ask for us to deliver lethal medicine to patients, but they can ask to withdraw care. The result can be the same.

My experience with Transplant spoke to me. I talked to Edward's mother about what I had learned about tragedy, from other lives, and the meaning that comes with it. I did something the hospital and my profession forbade. I shared with her that, if she asked me to take out the brain catheter, the last flame of life in her son's reptilian brain would succumb to the brain pressures created by undrained brain fluid. Removing the catheter would, essentially, let him go. This wasn't euthanasia. We wouldn't be administering a fatal dose but withdrawing one of the foreign things keeping Edward's brain alive. A breathing machine and medicinal drips would still keep his body alive. I told his mother that by doing this her son could save seven other lives.

If this was done, it might allow her to extract some meaning from the cruellest fate, the loss of a child. Maybe Edward's mother and fiancée would avoid pathological grief, a chronic, persistent, disabling grief that overtakes daily life. Through the alchemy of transplant medicine, her wrenching loss could turn to rebirth for others, new life for people on the edge. Finding meaning in terrible circumstances is why some cancer patients want to enroll in early-stage clinical trials. They want to advance medicine, to help others, even as their own fate is sealed. It's why others, like Jane, offer their bodies for rapid autopsy.

David Kessler, who collaborated with Elisabeth Kübler-Ross, believes there should be a sixth stage of grief: meaning. Kessler was already an expert on grief when it struck home: his son died of an accidental drug overdose at the age of twenty-one. Kessler believes that only by finding meaning can grief become something more peaceful, hopeful even. The same is true of any loss. Finding meaning in trauma, tragedy or heartbreak can be what keeps us going, and meaning can come from many places.

As creators of our own narrative selves, we also have the final say on the 'who am I?' question. Some manage to answer this question after they're dead, writing their epilogue posthumously, bequeathing assets to their favourite causes. Jane donated her tumours for research. Even though her cancer outlived her, her story continues, her cells propagating and driving scientific discovery and future medicine. Legacy.

Edward's mother asked me to pull the brain catheter. Her child was hanging off a cliff by a branch, and she asked me to cut that branch and let him fall. I broke the rules and guided her through a narrative that still makes my stomach knot up. But she also made a request, something unexpected and unheard of. Edward was her only child and the last of a generation. She wanted to have a chance at having grandchildren. So I made arrangements to assist a urology resident in removing his testicles as the non-negotiable part of her consent to organ donation, in the hope that IVF could enable his fiancée to have Edward's child. I never came to know if they went forward with their plans, but I felt at peace for having tried to offer some hope and possibility in their tragedy.

As I walked out of the operating theatre with the testicles, Greg happened to be washing his hands outside a different operating room. We looked at each other and paused for a moment. We didn't speak then, and we have never spoken about it since. The cooler I'd carried before had contained replacement parts that would save lives. This cooler had the potential to create life.

Edward's funeral was held in a small beach town. His fiancée and mother invited me, and during the ceremony his mother thanked 'Dr Jandial'. Edward's mother, who was only in her forties, was calling me 'Doctor', looking up to me as a neurosurgeon. But, to me, it felt like stolen valour. I had failed to save a young man, her son, after a brain haemorrhage, and here she was, at his funeral, thanking me. I felt like a pilot who had bailed out at the last minute in a crash that had taken her son. I was thanked by the grieving for trying my best. At the time, I didn't know what to do with my emotions. I felt at home nowhere and exiled everywhere after that experience. I hadn't shared it with anyone at the hospital. The only time

I'd felt at home was during that defining late-night conversation with Edward's mother in the ICU, when I wasn't a physician or even a surgeon. I was just me.

When I opened the path to brain death for Edward, I'd tried to offer his mother a way to make some sense out of madness, out of the randomness of the tragedy. I'd done it out of my allegiance to the patient and his loved ones, not to medicine or surgery or the ethics committee or the corporate hospital. I had tipped off his mother so that she might find some peace by facilitating brain death in a way that left parts of her son salvageable and plantable in other human beings. Saving his testicles made me feel decent for having gone the extra distance, that I was more than a surgeon. I was someone who could find meaning in death and offer a different kind of healing to those suffering loss.

Loss and life are linked inextricably. It is the very depth of those bonds and attachments that makes the loss so disruptive, so deeply painful. It is impossible to live without experiencing loss. And when I have seen it pierce the lives of patients and loved ones, I have witnessed humanity at both its most raw and its most robust.

Grieving, if you let it serve you, can open the doors to remembrance. It is being able to find some meaning in the life that was lived that allows us to make some sense of the senseless. The loss is no less real, but the burden becomes one we are able to bear.

10.

Life

Locked-in syndrome is more like a decapitation than a medical condition. The guillotine falls not at the neck but at the mouth, through the hinge of your jaw and through your brainstem. Your thinking and emotional brain remain intact, isolated, an island in an inert sea. All the voluntary muscles below the eyes are paralysed. You are left with the ability to see and blink. Nothing else.

With locked-in syndrome, you need everything the ICU has to offer: strong medicines in your blood, a machine pumping air in and out of your lungs through a hose in your throat, a bag squeezing viscous off-white pureed food directly into your stomach from a puncture in your abdominal wall. The only thing you don't need are lubricating eyedrops. Your lacrimal glands can still produce tears.

There is no cure for locked-in syndrome. Your skull becomes your sanctuary and your prison, your final refuge. Because there is no obvious response to verbal or even painful stimuli, in the distant past patients with locked-in syndrome were thought to be in a coma. Thrust a needle, and they don't react. Slice their chest, and they lie restful. Seemingly insensate. What they feel is concealed, except for those tears, but tears can happen reflexively. Emotional tears have a different composition.

Locked-in syndrome can be caused by a stroke in the brainstem, diseases such as multiple sclerosis or by rare surgical complications. In this case, my surgery was the cause.

This patient had a slowly growing meningioma inside the base of her cranial vault. The ball of tissue that had grown was benign, but that didn't mean it wasn't dangerous. Barricaded by the skull like a creeping plant blocked by a brick wall, it did what it could. It grew upwards, downwards, almost as though it was attempting to escape the skull entirely, heading for its escape hatch through the beautifully geometric oval exit at the bottom of the skull called the foramen magnum. Before that liberation, it had knuckled into the pliable brainstem, the path of least resistance.

The brainstem sits beneath the brain's hemispheres like the stalk of a large mushroom; the cap is the meandering ridges of the cerebral hemispheres. The brainstem funnels the signals between the brain and body. It also houses the reticular activating system, or RAS, a light switch for consciousness.

This patient's tumour dented these delicate controls in its glacial expansion. As a result, parts of her body were already losing the descending commands.

When the patient first walked into my clinic, it looked like she was drunk. Her movements would soon be so demolished that her whole body would be flaccid. A wheelchair would be an impossible challenge.

The tumour had grown slowly, glacially, over decades, unrelenting. Although it was benign, it would grow and be partially cut out, return and be radiated, return and be cut again. Because of its proximity to the brainstem, the tumour couldn't be completely removed. Each time, the patient would enjoy brief windows without further disability. Each time, it grew closer to the brainstem, meaning that each surgery cut out the tumour ever more partially – until it had her brainstem in a vice. Three surgeries by two other surgeons across America had stemmed the tide for almost a decade.

She was now in LA. She said, 'I know you can't get it all. I just need another debulking to shave down my enemy.' Over the years, she had come to know the foe within, and told me, 'It doesn't know any better,' strangely absolving it of guilt.

Before, she'd wanted the surgery so she could live long enough for her kids to be out of the house. Now, she was no longer under that pressure. This time, she said, 'I'm doing this just for me.' She had been operated on by senior reputable people, but they had since died or stopped practising, so she came to see me.

She asked for my advice. We talked briefly about the risks. This wasn't her first rodeo. We discussed the possibility of a devastating stroke. As it is so rare, locked-in syndrome never came up. For her surgery, I suggested the shortest route to the tumour: through her mouth. This was more dangerous but had an advantage. It was virgin territory and hadn't been operated on before. The other approaches were already scarred down heavily from prior operations. She agreed, and that's the approach I took.

To begin the surgery, I placed a retractor in the patient's mouth to open it wide. I stood by her right shoulder, a microscope descending from the ceiling, and cut through the back of the throat, a vertical slice. My cut ran parallel to the brainstem's fibres deeper beneath, those clusters of magical neurons that make us breathe, gag, cough, even wake up. In this case, perfect meant shaving out what I could to buy the patient time. The surgery was going smoothly, as far as I could tell.

The surgery had taken place at the base of the skull, which is penetrated by four arteries coming up off the heart: two in the front, which you can feel on either side of your throat, called the carotids; and two which snake through your cervical spine, the verte-brals, entering the skull and converging into a single trunk, the basilar artery.

The basilar artery feeds the brainstem. The brain-stem has no redundant tissue. Every square millimetre does something measurable. Every square millimetre matters, unlike in the cortical canopy, where there is a lot of crossover and redundancy. Damage to even its smaller, hair-thin tributaries can leave one wrecked: never able to eat, never breathing independently, never conscious. Remarkable are the features of the unique landscape the basilar irrigates.

I don't remember hitting the tributaries off the basilar artery, wispy arteries called 'perforators', notorious because they are both indispensable and exquisitely frail. The lightest caress makes them spasm shut, cutting off the blood supply.

The most critical parts of our bodies and brains usually have some redundant extra flow from two or more arteries. There's one exception where there aren't two vessels, and the exception is responsible for the most fundamental part of our existence – consciousness. The part of the brain that turns our lights on – or off. There is an immediacy to an injury to this area of the ancient brain. The brainstem is unforgiving; it relies only on these bizarre, tiny dead-end arteries which have no help from neighbouring vessels.

Consciousness doesn't ignite from the undulating surface of the brain, the canopy of neurons, where lies the source of art and science, humour and love. None of this is allowed to fire unless a certain spark of consciousness shivers upwards from the brainstem's primal gate. Without that, nothing else is even given a chance. The *Mona Lisa* and the Sistine Chapel sit in the dark.

After surgery, I thought this patient was comatose.

We did a basic and quick brain scan, but it didn't show any injury to tissue that could explain her condition. But the dark centre of her eyes, her pupils, briskly closed under bright light. And then a thought surfaced in my mind, and probably hers. I started to wonder if she was locked in. I ordered an EEG and the test showed the brainwaves of someone who was awake. They weren't the rapid-fire gamma waves of someone stressed out but the alpha waves of someone calm.

The fibres carrying the southbound and northbound signals from the brainstem aren't intermixed, they are distinct, like lanes on opposing sides of a highway. What the injury did was take out nearly all the southbound lanes, from her mouth down. The only functional southbound lane remaining was above the damage. This lane exited to the eyeballs. Many or even most of the northbound lanes remained intact, which meant that the patient could feel pain but she couldn't express it. She was left only with the ability to see and blink. That's it. Absolutely nothing else moved in her body. Vision and hearing were her access to the world and our only way to access her inconceivable inner world.

In *The Count of Monte Cristo*, Alexander Dumas describes the look of someone with locked-in syndrome as being 'like the distant gleam of a candle which a traveller sees by night across some desert place'. Concentrated in his eyes, he added, were:

All the activity, address, force, and intelligence which were formerly diffused over his whole body; and so although the movement of the arm, the sound of the voice, and the agility of the body, were wanting, the speaking eye sufficed for all.

We quickly assembled teams of consultants to communicate with the patient, and a visual placard was set up with letters on a card. We ran our fingers over the letters, and she blinked when a letter was selected. She blinked in doublets. Blink-blink. I insisted she give us this double blink to show it was no accident. A single blink can be reflexive.

Blinking as we moved through the alphabet, she resembled a contestant in a strange version of the American game show *Wheel of Fortune*, forming words and phrases one vowel and consonant at a time. Her eyes were the tiny windows to her consciousness. It was as though she were trapped in a house and could communicate only by controlling the blinds. She was the miner buried deep below the surface, tapping out her intentions.

What happens to the notion of self when the self is locked in, limited to the mind, constrained, squeezed into the smallest confines allowing for consciousness? The French journalist Jean-Dominique Bauby suffered a massive injury and awoke with locked-in syndrome at a hospital on the coast near Normandy. He was forty-three at the time. He likened his

condition to being trapped in a diving bell. Letter by
letter, he wrote a book, *The Diving Bell and the Butterfly: A Memoir of Life in Death.* The butterfly was his
mind, with its ability to take wing and transport him
beyond the cage his body had become. The neurobiologist Santiago Ramón y Cajal, who revealed that
neurons communicate with one another but never
physically touch, also compared the mind to butterflies:

> Like the entomologist in search of colorful butter-
> flies, my attention has chased in the gardens of the
> grey matter cells with delicate and elegant shapes,
> the mysterious butterflies of the soul, whose beating
> of wings may one day reveal to us the secrets of the
> mind.

In Bauby's first-person account of locked-in syndrome, he shares the limits of the butterflies' abilities
to transport him to other places and other times.

> I am fading away. Slowly but surely. Like the sailor
> who watches his home shore gradually disappear, I
> watch my past recede. My old life still burns within
> me, but more and more of it is reduced to the ashes
> of memory.

For those on the outside looking in, it may seem
that patients with chronic locked-in syndrome have

nothing to live for. The patients themselves typically disagree. Some find a meaning, a sense of well-being, from their 'internal' experiences. In fact, they rate their quality of life in the same range as age-matched healthy individuals. This surprises people, especially their caregivers, who rate their quality of life much lower than the patients do themselves.

Bauby did not shy away from the severe and often heartbreaking limitations of his condition, but he was still able to find joy. He wrote about the letters friends sent to his hospital, describing every-day life:

> Roses picked at dusk, the laziness of a rainy Sunday, a child crying himself to sleep. Capturing the moment, these small slices of life, these small gusts of happiness, move me more deeply than all the rest . . . I hoard all these letters like a treasure. One day I hope to fasten them to a half-mile-long streamer, to float in the wind like a banner to the glory of friendship. It will keep the vultures at bay.

My patient had signed all the legal paperwork. She had acknowledged the myriad risks of surgery, just as anyone undergoing even the most benign procedure accepts the chance of serious injury or death. Even 'Acts of God' such as earthquakes are covered. Most patients barely read the forms before they sign. Unlike many patients, my patient had been acutely aware of the dangers of her surgery. She knew the edge she was teetering on.

Now, she had no control over her body, but she could blink her wishes. We talked about her discharge to a nursing home that takes people on ventilators, we talked about where she lived and how to find one close to her home. She still had agency. She still had some control over what was left of her life, just as Jane had directed her days with cancer. With this, she could extract meaning. Out of the blue, she spelled D-O-N-A-T-E, and I was perplexed. Donate what? H-E-A-R-T. And then she spelled L-U-N-G-S. To leave no doubt, she spelled it out, literally: D-O-N-A-T-E. O-R-G-A-N-S. W-A-N-T T-O B-E O-R-G-A-N D-O-N-O-R.

Most people whose organs are 'harvested' have made their wishes known prior to catastrophe, or their relatives have made the decision if they are brain dead and deemed too far gone for recovery. Blinking her will to donate her organs was a clinical scenario that had never been described before.

Once she'd made it clear she wanted to donate her organs, the entire ICU was overwhelmed by what we were witnessing: her search for purpose and meaning in the midst of devastating circumstances. I thought of Edward's mother from nearly a decade before. Meaning in tragedy. Purpose in suffering.

The day after she expressed those wishes to be an organ donor, we assumed it would be in the distant future, but we were wrong. She was driving me to a place I couldn't have imagined. We ran the questions again: What's your name? What year is it? What city are you in? The process was time-consuming. Blink blink . . . pause . . . blink blink . . . pause . . . blink blink. The resolution of those eyeballs, locked in the socket, unmoving, because it's a different cranial nerve than the one used by the eyelids for blinking.

After reiterating her desire to donate organs, the patient said that she wanted to set up withdrawal of care. This is something a close member of the family usually does, not the patient themselves. Do you want us to remove the breathing machine? Y-E-S. Do you want to stay on the breathing machine? N-O. Will you live or die if we remove the machine? Will you live or die if we keep the machine? Are you afraid of death? Or dying? Despite her glazed-over face, without any muscular contraction, her eyes were so calm, as if she had been waiting for me to finally come to realize that it was her right, her life, her opportunity to escape from the cage. The final question. What are you afraid of? She responded: L-I-V-I-N-G.

Euthanasia is illegal, but patients do have the right to sign documents detailing under which circumstances there should be cessation of care. We all have that right, but it's established before you're on 'life support'. The directives are carried out in hospitals for patients who are not conscious, and the wish is certainly not made by the patient themselves.

I'd slept well the night before because I'd felt that I was doing the right thing. I had no doubt about what the patient wanted, and what she wanted did not conflict with my *self*, how I viewed my purpose in the world. Since we were on this inexorable ride to something unsalvageable, it didn't feel like failure. Even so, I woke up that morning with a strange frisson of profound anxiety. I was no longer sure about anything. The appointment was set for noon on a Sunday. I didn't want the hospital to be in the midst of a busy weekday for this.

The day before, I had communicated with her again, alone. I apologized, and she came back at me: S-O-R-R-Y . . . W-H-Y. Over an hour of conversation at the pace of using one key at a time on an old typewriter, we connected. It was an indescribable conversation. Sign language with blinks, my finger caressing the board left to right across the lines of letters. Waiting for a blink-blink and starting to anticipate and autocorrect. After T-H-, the options were narrower, but still open. They, them . . . thank you.

She apologized to me for bringing such a complicated case to my doorstep. I got the feeling she was waiting for me to process my grief, waiting for me to catch up with her. She had been engaging with this slow but relentless threat on her most basic life functions for years. Maybe she had already gone through innumerable strata of grief. She blinked and made it clear through her message that this was not a frantic Morse code SOS from a sinking ship but something quite different – not save our souls but release my soul. Our conversation was unlike anything I'd experienced before or since. The pace of the back and forth was strangely peaceful. Waiting for her to blink at each letter slowed time, required me to step off my cadence. The experience was meditative.

On the day she had chosen to let go, I made a conscious effort not to dress or look differently than I had in the weeks past. I rarely wear a white coat and had thought about wearing one that day but decided that would break from the ritual. It might create anxiety in her. I didn't want her to think I was treating this day as a rarefied moment. I didn't want her to think I was having second thoughts, but I was. This was, in essence, physician-assisted suicide. This was so different to the more than hundreds I had withdrawn care on, in each case based on directives that had been written by the patient in advance or given by family. This was a completely conscious patient asking me to cut the rope.

The nurses joined me in preparing my patient to let go of her life. I would guide and remove large tubes and shafts so that when her family said their goodbyes they could have their loved one looking as much like herself as possible before we took out the one, crucial tube at the end. The tubes look like parachutes when the patient is alive and fighting for life. When the patient surrenders, the foreign objects look like the residues of failure. When most of my patients reach their end, the dangling morphine is the exit ramp. Our gentle nudge that lets everyone know that there is no turning back. We document in the notes that the increased morphine is for pain, but we all know that morphine also results in respiratory depression and a quicker, calmer exit. But she refused.

She tired of looking at the ceiling. She was limited in her peripheral vision and she wanted to be sitting up a little. We put a strap under her arms and a small pillow either side of her neck so her head would be upright. And now, she was braced and looking forward.

At her left bedside, I held the alphabet placard in front of her and moved my fingers across the flat letters. Braille for me with my eyes open. Everyone else did what they could to project an air of composure. I caressed the letters and we went through the questions a final time. Do you want us to remove the breathing machine? Y-E-S. Do you want to stay on the breathing machine? N-O.

I didn't know where this was hitting my brain. Braille takes finger sensations and sends them to the derelict vision region of the brain in the blind. Did this visual perception send shivers to the sensation parts of my brain, my fingers, the same hands that had put her here? Did they send electric quivers to my insula because I could feel the sinking feeling in my stomach?

Extubation is the removal of a thick plastic tube from the lungs, just above where the trachea splits left and right like an upside-down trunk. For her, the extubation couldn't elicit the usual cough; the scratching plastic triggers the cough and gag reflex at the back of the throat. But her eyes would tear when the tube was removed. Looking back, I wish I could have collected her tears and sent them off to the lab to look for pain, isolation, grief. Her exit would be wide awake.

Her eyes were alert and calm. No fright. None that I could see. It wasn't the distraught look I've seen in moments of crisis for patients and their families. This time, I was the one needing consolation. This time, I was the one with fright in my eyes. I was shaken. This was different to all the other times I've said goodbye to patients. I wanted to know what she was feeling so I'd know what I was allowed to feel.

Her body wouldn't object. Lost cough and gag reflexes meant that sedating medicine could be turned off. It had to be that way. She wanted it that way. It was critical in establishing that she was her true self.

And when she let go, she gave a salvo of double blinks. Never just blinking once, probably to reassure me. And then not blinking at all.

+++++++++++++++++++

In that moment, I felt our shared humanity, and something else – that I had so much to learn. About life, and about myself. About who I had become and who I could still be. Lessons about life, loss and rules for survival are everywhere: in the individual cells in our brains, in our minds, in my patients, in the surgery, in my practice, operating at the margins of life and death, hope and hopelessness. Life at its edges and depths also reveals its heights. That no tragedy or triumph is forever. We are new every day in our brains and, if we try – in our minds.

Brain cells have rules for their survival, developing into special cell types that automatically coalesce, from a mysterious force drawing together the components of our brains, as if we were meant to be part of something greater. Individual neurons reach out not just towards neighbours but across vast ensembles, creating forests with trillions of overlapping branches and producing symphonies of brainwaves from a design that favours greater complexity, kinship and possibility.

Our minds, too, push us towards survival. To cope, we strive towards a coherent sense of self, balancing the cognitive and the emotional, all to make us better equipped for threat, trauma, pressure, performance and loss. Struggles endured and overcome inoculate us for future struggles. Habits of thought, care and discipline in our thinking can harness emotions without becoming harnessed by them. Emotional regulation is not the lack of emotion, rather it is emotion at its finest and most lush. This realization can actually change the very nature of the flesh from which it arises, leaving us with an understanding of how we are anchored in biology, but not imprisoned by it.

Patients have their own methods of survival. Not every patient suffers well, yet some are triumphant, accessing human nature at its most transcendent, their lives punctuated by growth in trying circumstances. For these people, their diagnosis did not put their life on hold. Not blinded by death, or dying, they are able to find their true priorities, casting aside distractions that had long encumbered them. Their ability to see themselves in a new light is their most important transformation, whether it's gradual or comes as an epiphany.

In the operating theatre, I have my own rules of survival. I've come to savour the craft of surgery, knowing that what matters is not dazzling manoeuvres or groundbreaking operations but the lives patients have when they wake up. Being at my best means engaging emotions in the moment and balancing them, breathing through any fear into a flow state. True performance in the operating theatre means performing in a way that is true to myself.

I have learned many lessons on survival through my life. Mostly from my patients. They have shown me that the evolution of our interior life is not a constant process but fluctuates in and out of equilibrium;

it is both vulnerable and resilient. That introspection and imagination allow us not to be solely defined by our origins but by our direction, too.

More and more, I am amazed by their gratitude, often thinking to myself: for what? I should thank them for graciously allowing me to be a part of their most intense and intimate moments. And permitting me to learn from their trials: to not wait for calamity to provide clarity. The goal is not to become imperturbable. Savour the joys and create a process for coping through difficult times.

I thank my patients for trusting me. For teaching me. For so long, I thought myself to be a spectator of their lives. But I have been touched by their journey. Informed by it. Transformed by it.

Acknowledgements

Venetia Butterfield gave me this opportunity and believed I was capable of more. She has simply changed the trajectory of my life. I am beyond indebted and deeply grateful. And it was fun too.

Mel Berger brought me into the publishing ecosystem and is closer to a mentor than an agent. Fiona Baird has been a great liaison with Penguin Random House.

Lydia Yadi joined the project and has added momentum and finesse. She has been a delight to work with. Amy McWalters gave thoughtful feedback, and Sarah Day has enhanced the book further.

Julia Murday led an amazing campaign to publicize my first book with Emma Finnigan, and I look forward to working with them on this one as well.

David Martin has been more than a collaborator during the back-and-forth construction of this book: his intelligence and kindness gave me consolation while working in the hospitals in 2020.

And, of course, to my patients, who have enriched my life by allowing me to share in theirs: thank you.